Defining Psychopathology
in the 21st Century

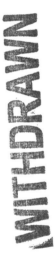

Defining Psychopathology in the 21st Century

DSM-V and Beyond

Edited by

John E. Helzer, M.D.

James J. Hudziak, M.D.

American Psychopathological Association

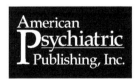

Washington, D.C.
London, England

Manufactured in the United States of America on acid-free paper
06 05 04 03 02   5 4 3 2 1
First Edition

American Psychiatric Publishing, Inc.
1400 K Street, N.W.
Washington, DC 20005
www.appi.org

Library of Congress Cataloging-in-Publication Data
Defining psychopathology in the 21st century : DSM-V and beyond / edited by John E. Helzer, James J. Hudziak.—1st ed.
    p. ; cm.
    Includes bibliographical references and index.
    ISBN 1-58562-063-7 (alk. paper)
    1. Mental illness—Classification—Congresses. 2. Mental illness—Longitudinal studies—Congresses. 3. Mental illness—Diagnosis—Congresses. I. Title: Defining psychopathology in the twenty first century. II. Helzer, John E. III. Hudziak, James J.
    [DNLM: 1. Mental Disorders—classification—Congresses. 2. Diagnostic Imaging—Congresses. 3. Longitudinal Studies—Congresses. 4. Mental Disorders—diagnosis—Congresses. WM 15 D313 2002]
    RC455.2.C4 D44 2002
    616.89′001′2—dc21   2001053745

British Library Cataloguing in Publication Data
A CIP record is available from the British Library.

One of the privileges of a prestigious university is the opportunity to know and be influenced by great men like Sam Guze. His death is a loss for the profession and a personal loss for those of us he taught. We are grateful that the Millennial meeting of the American Psychopathological Association provided us the opportunity to give Sam the Joseph Zubin Award, the only award our association confers that Sam had not been honored with. Sam richly deserved the award, but it was a pittance compared to our debt to him.

JEH
JJH

Contents

Contributors

Thomas M. Achenbach, Ph.D.
Professor of Psychiatry
  and Psychology
University of Vermont
Burlington, Vermont

Kelly N. Botteron, M.D.
Assistant Professor
Departments of Psychiatry
  and Radiology
Washington University School
  of Medicine
St. Louis, Missouri

Stephen L. Buka, Sc.D.
Associate Professor
Departments of Maternal and
  Child Health and Epidemiology
Harvard School of Public Health
Boston, Massachusetts

Wayne C. Drevets, M.D.
Associate Professor
Departments of Psychiatry
  and Radiology
University of Pittsburgh
Pittsburgh, Pennsylvania
Chief, Mood and Anxiety Disorders
  Neuroimaging Section
National Institute of Mental Health
National Institutes of Health
Bethesda, Maryland

Jane Epstein, M.D.
Assistant Professor of Psychiatry
Weill Cornell Medical College
New York, New York

Stephen V. Faraone, Ph.D.
Associate Professor of Psychiatry
Harvard Medical School
    Department of Psychiatry
    at the Massachusetts Mental
    Health Center
Director of Research
Pediatric Psychopharmacology
    Unit, Psychiatry Service
Massachusetts General Hospital
Boston, Massachusetts

Stephen E. Gilman, Sc.D.
Research Fellow
Departments of Maternal and Child
    Health and Health and Social
    Behavior
Harvard School of Public Health
Boston, Massachusetts

John E. Helzer, M.D.
Professor of Psychiatry
Health Behavior Research Center
University of Vermont School
    of Medicine
Burlington, Vermont

James J. Hudziak, M.D.
Associate Professor of Psychiatry and
    Medicine (Division of Human
    Medical Genetics)
Director of Child Psychiatry
University of Vermont College of
    Medicine
Burlington, Vermont

Nancy Isenberg, M.D., M.P.H.
Assistant Professor of Neurology
Seton Hall University and
    New Jersey Neuroscience Institute
JFK Medical Center
Edison, New Jersey

Peter S. Jensen, M.D.
Professor of Psychiatry
Department of Psychiatry
Columbia University College
    of Physicians and Surgeons
New York, New York

Robert E. Kendell, M.D.
Honorary Professor of Psychiatry
University of Edinburgh
Scotland, United Kingdom

Robert F. Krueger, Ph.D.
Assistant Professor
Department of Psychology
University of Minnesota–Twin
    Cities
Minneapolis, Minnesota

Kathleen R. Merikangas, Ph.D.
Professor of Epidemiology and
    Public Health, Psychiatry, and
    Psychology
Yale University School of
    Medicine
New Haven, Connecticut
Senior Investigator
National Institute of Mental Health
Bethesda, Maryland

William E. Narrow, M.D., M.P.H.
Director, Psychopathology Research
    Program
American Psychiatric Institute for
    Research and Education
Washington, D.C.

Darrel A. Regier, M.D., M.P.H.
Executive Director
American Psychiatric Institute for
    Research and Education
Washington, D.C.

John S. Searles, Ph.D.
Research Assistant Professor
Health Behavior Research Center
University of Vermont School
    of Medicine
Burlington, Vermont

David Silbersweig, M.D.
Assistant Professor of Psychiatry,
    Neurology, and Neuroscience
Weill Cornell Medical College
New York, New York

Robert L. Spitzer, M.D.
Professor of Psychiatry
Department of Psychiatry
Columbia University
The New York State Psychiatric
  Institute
New York, New York

Emily Stern, M.D.
Assistant Professor of Radiology
  in Psychiatry
Assistant Professor of Radiology
Weill Cornell Medical College
New York, New York

Ming T. Tsuang, M.D., Ph.D.
Stanley Cobb Professor of Psychiatry
Harvard Medical School
Director, Harvard Institute of Psychiatric
  Epidemiology and Genetics
Head, Harvard Department of Psychiatry
  at Massachusetts Mental Health Center
Boston, Massachusetts

Jerome C. Wakefield, D.S.W., Ph.D.
Professor, School of Social Work
  and Institute for Health, Health Care
  Policy, and Aging Research
Rutgers University
New Brunswick, New Jersey

Preface

The American Psychopathological Association (APPA) has a rich history of interest in and contributions to the taxonomies that have been used in medicine to define psychopathology. From Adolf Meyer to commonsense psychiatry to current members' contributions refining the DSM through the use of basic and clinical research, members of the APPA have often taken the lead in the development of psychiatric taxonomies. This volume, coordinated from the annual meeting in 2000, "Defining Psychopathology in the 21st Century," is devoted to this topic. The hope for the millennium meeting and for this resulting volume is that they will challenge debate about the tensions between the convenience of a clinically derived categorical taxonomy and the growing research need for more empirically derived, dimensional systems. The author of Chapter 1 of this volume, Robert Kendell, who wrote brilliantly about the need for categories in his book *The Role of Diagnosis in Psychiatry*, was also challenging us to think more dimensionally as far back as the 1970s. Obviously, this is hardly a new issue in psychopathology. However, there is growing concern that broad categories of illness are insufficient to serve new research needs, perhaps most acutely in genetics research.

Within this text are 15 chapters devoted to the goal of developing approaches to classification that will lead to more accurate diagnoses and treatments for our patients and to a broader range of taxonomic options for research. We have devoted 4 chapters to "Definitional Tensions," in which among other topics, Dr. Kendell presents a list of five criteria for a better taxonomy. It appears certain that the advances in neuroimaging will forever change the conceptualization of "disorder" in psychiatry. Thus, we committed a number of chapters to the contribution of imaging studies to improving our diagnostic approaches. Too little attention has been paid to the developmental/longitudinal contribution to diagnostic considerations; hence, we included meaningful discussions of collecting data over time. With the publication of the human genome sequence and the assurance that a large number of the genes yet to be defined will be genes that contribute to behavior, we devoted 4 chapters to the consideration of genetic epidemiology in subjects of all ages and both genders to develop, as Dr. Faraone argues, "a genetically meaningful taxonomy."

This was both a sweet and sad conference for us. Our science has never been more exciting or important. We were able to honor two of our members with awards that recognize their long contribution to the field and to the APPA. Dr. Stephen Faraone presented Dr. Ming T. Tsuang with the Paul Hoch Award, recognizing his lifelong contribution to psychiatric genetics. In his presentation and in his chapter in this volume, Dr. Tsuang argued for using our new methodologies in the consideration of treating subsyndromal or preschizophrenia, a taxonomic condition he defines as "schizotaxia."

For many of us, this was the last time we spent with Dr. Samuel B. Guze, who was honored with this year's Joseph Zubin Award. Dr. Guze and his work have touched almost all members of the APPA, and it is for this reason that we mark his passing by dedicating this volume to him.

Acknowledgments

We would like to acknowledge two individuals who were crucial to the successful completion of this volume. First is Michele Comette, our Editorial Assistant. Michele added the work on this book to her already full plate as Research Assistant in Dr. Helzer's center and her assistantship with his other editorial responsibilities. Her efficiency, energy, and organizational skills kept the project on track. Her good humor helped editors and authors retain theirs.

Second is Pamela Harley, Managing Editor at American Psychiatric Publishing, Inc. Pam's experience and guidance were vital in negotiating the myriad details of coordinating a multiauthored work with a major publishing house. She performed this legerdemain under the considerable pressure of our self-imposed, tight publication deadlines.

Finally, we would like to acknowledge the American Psychopathological Association (APPA) for the opportunity to organize and conduct the
millennial APPA meeting and to publish this volume. Through its nearly
100 years of existence, the APPA has remained a vibrant organization. Its
annual meeting is an outstanding forum for the lively exchange of scientific
ideas. The many scientists who regularly attend consider it indispensable
to their continuing education as researchers in psychopathology.

John E. Helzer, M.D.
James J. Hudziak, M.D.

PART I DEFINITIONAL TENSIONS

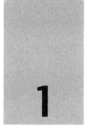

1

Five Criteria for an Improved Taxonomy of Mental Disorders

Robert E. Kendell, M.D.

Before the prospects for a better taxonomy of mental disorders are discussed, it obviously has to be agreed what characteristics would make a new taxonomy in some way "better" than our present ones—essentially DSM-IV (American Psychiatric Association 1994) and the International Classification of Diseases (ICD-10; World Health Organization [WHO] 1992). I suggest that there are five main ways in which a new taxonomy might be regarded as an improvement. It might

1. be more comprehensive,
2. be easier to use,
3. deal better with the issue of "clinical significance,"
4. have higher reliability, or
5. have higher validity.

It has to be accepted from the outset, though, that different users may have differing views about what constitutes an improvement, because their needs are different. Research workers and clinicians will have different priorities and so too may specialists whose clinical practice is concentrated on a single class of disorders and generalists who treat a much wider range of patients.

COMPREHENSIVENESS AND EASE OF USE

The first two criteria are fairly easily dealt with. All classifications of disease tend to become more complex and comprehensive every time they are revised or with each new edition. This is partly because the range of conditions that clinicians are interested in or consulted about, and therefore need to classify, keeps expanding and partly because increasing experience and understanding of individual disorders often convinces clinicians that conditions are heterogenous and ought to be subdivided. In DSM-II, for example, behavior disorders of childhood and adolescence were covered in just two pages, and there was just one subcategory for all disorders of sleep (306.4) and another for all feeding disturbances (306.5) (American Psychiatric Association 1968). Indeed, the whole glossary weighed just 200 g, compared with the 1,050 g of DSM-III (American Psychiatric Association 1980) and the 1,320 g of DSM-IV.

The more detailed and comprehensive a classification becomes, the more complicated it is to use, particularly if it involves multiple axes and operational definitions. There is an immediate tension therefore between these first two criteria of improvement, and clinicians, research workers, specialists, and generalists are all likely to have different views about which criterion is more important. For the reasons I have alluded to, future classifications will tend to be more complicated and comprehensive than those we have now. It is essential therefore that the enthusiasts who design these classifications do not forget that most psychiatrists and clinical psychologists do not share their preoccupation with definitions and classification. Their sophisticated and painstakingly constructed glossaries will need to be accepted and used by ordinary clinicians, and this will probably require the simultaneous production of a simplified pocket edition.

CLINICAL SIGNIFICANCE

My third criterion concerns the issue of clinical significance, or handicap. The Epidemiologic Catchment Area and National Comorbidity Surveys (Kessler et al. 1994; Robins and Regier 1991), based on the definitions of DSM-III and DSM-III-R (American Psychiatric Association 1987) respectively, generated unexpectedly high prevalence rates for several disorders. This led to criticisms that these definitions were overinclusive and generating "false positives"—that many respondents who genuinely met the symptomatic criteria of the disorder in question were not significantly handicapped by their symptoms and should not therefore have been labeled as having a mental disorder. This problem was discussed by the task force responsible for DSM-IV, and a decision was made to add an additional "clinical significance" criterion to the definitions of nearly half of all Axis I and II disorders. This was a cumbersome strategy that has proved only partially successful in eliminating false positives.

Spitzer and Wakefield (1999) recently discussed the problem in some detail. They argued that a better solution would be either to revise the definitions of individual disorders to guarantee that the combinations of symptoms required are sufficient to guarantee a significant impairment of function or to add a criterion that excludes normal reactions to psychosocial stress. In my view this is a better solution, although I agree with Kendler (1999) that it would not deal with all aspects of the problem. For one thing, removing a redundant stipulation from the definition of over 100 disorders would produce a welcome reduction in the size and complexity of the glossary as a whole. It also would be well worthwhile revising the basic DSM definition of mental disorder in light of Wakefield's (1992) cogent analysis of the concept. Wakefield argued that the concept of disease or disorder—whether mental or physical—has two components. It requires both a biological dysfunction, meaning the failure of an internal mechanism to perform a natural function for which it was designed, and evidence of what he calls *harm* and the WHO (1980) rather more appropriately calls *handicap*. (WHO defines *handicap* as "a disadvantage, for a given individual, resulting from an impairment or a disability, that limits or prevents the fulfillment of a role that is normal [depending on age, sex, and social and cultural factors] for that individual" [1980, p. 29].) *Dysfunction,* Wakefield argued, is a value-free scientific term, whereas harm or handicap is dependent on both environmental circumstances and cultural attitudes. Having struggled myself (Kendell 1975, 1986) to decide whether disease and disorder are better regarded as normative concepts based on value judgments or as value-free scientific terms, I am impressed by Wakefield's argument that both elements are necessarily involved. More important, in the present context, his argument that a biological dysfunction and a handicap are both essential elements of mental disorders implies that any additional criterion of clinical significance is redundant.

This implies that mental disorders such as depressive episode and generalized anxiety disorder must be defined in a way that associates them with significant handicap for most people in most common environmental settings. It does not mean, however, that every individual who meets criteria for these disorders has to be significantly handicapped. Not all people with diabetes, for example, are significantly harmed, or handicapped, by their disorder, even in the absence of treatment. However, they are at increased risk of several disabling complications and of premature death. It is important to remember, too, that Axis V of DSM-IV already provides—by a rating of 90 or more on the Global Assessment of Functioning Scale—a means of recording whether the disorder in question significantly handicaps the individual in his or her present environment.

The fact that some psychiatric disorders have a surprisingly high prevalence in the general population does not necessarily mean that they have been inappropriately defined. Some people do regard it as absurd that at any given time 10%–15% of the population is suffering from a mental disorder and that nearly 30% may do so in the course of a year; however, I believe that this reaction is related to the stigma associated with mental illness. To these people, mental illness is a terrible and rather shameful affliction that, mercifully, affects only other people. The suggestion that a substantial proportion of the population has mental disorders threatens to impinge uncomfortably on their families and friends as well as themselves. It was demonstrated long ago, much to everyone's surprise at that time, that most people have troublesome physical symptoms most of the time. A community survey of the inhabitants of two south London boroughs in 1971 found that 95% of respondents considered themselves to have been "unwell" in some respect in the previous 14 days (Wadsworth et al. 1971). A similar survey in another English city found that only 5% of respondents had been completely symptom free over a similar period and that 9% claimed to have had more than six different symptoms during that period (Dunnell and Cartwright 1972). If physical disorders are so common—and no one doubts any longer that they are—there is no reason why psychiatric disorders should not be equally common, and it would be a big mistake, both scientifically and politically, to change our definitions in order to reduce their apparent prevalence. It would be even more ill advised to incorporate "need for treatment" into the definition, for what is *capable* of being treated successfully may quickly change and what is deemed to *merit* treatment is influenced by social, political, and economic forces.

RELIABILITY

My fourth criterion is high reliability. The reliability of most of the 200 categories of mental disorder listed in DSM-III was far higher than that of the corresponding categories in DSM-II because nearly all of them had an operational definition that specified unambiguously which combinations of symptoms and other characteristics were and were not sufficient to justify that diagnosis. The DSM-III Task Force also carried out extensive field trials, involving over 12,000 patients and 550 clinicians, in an attempt to ensure that ambiguous definitions were identified and reworded, and in the final field trials the task force achieved an average kappa coefficient in adult patients of 0.72 for Axis I disorders and 0.64 for Axis II disorders. This was the most important reason why DSM-III was, eventually, almost universally regarded as a far better and more useful taxonomy than any of its predecessors and why all of its successors—DSM-III-R, DSM-IV, DSM-IV-TR, and ICD-10—have provided operational definitions and have achieved comparable levels of reliability.

I would argue therefore that the battle to achieve acceptably high reliability has been won. Future taxonomies of mental disorders will almost certainly provide operational definitions for all, or nearly all, of their categories and achieve the same, or slightly higher, reliability as that of DSM-III. Although it will continue to be essential to test the reliability of all new definitions and to remove or reword ambiguous elements in them, it can probably be taken for granted that this will be done. Higher reliability is not, therefore, going to be the crucial feature that makes some future taxonomy demonstrably better than its predecessors. From now on, improvements in reliability will be modest and localized or secondary to a fundamental change in the nature of the defining characteristics of mental disorders.

VALIDITY

The last and crucial issue is that of validity. Indeed, reliability is important primarily because it establishes a ceiling for validity. The lower the reliability of a diagnostic category, the lower its validity necessarily becomes. (The converse, of course, is not true. Reliability can be high while validity remains trivial, and in such a situation high reliability is of little value.)

Reliability is easily measured. Validity is more nebulous, although the more important correlates a diagnostic category has over and above its defining characteristics, the less likely its validity will be questioned. Psychologists are accustomed to distinguishing several different kinds of validity—construct, concurrent, content, predictive, and so on. Although these are useful distinctions in many settings, in the context of clinical medicine statements about diagnostic validity are essentially statements about predictive power and hence about practical utility. The more information a diagnosis provides about outcome and response to treatment—and thus about which treatments are appropriate—the higher its validity and the greater its utility.

There is an old axiom that the art of taxonomy consists of "carving nature at the joints," which is an elegant way of saying that optimal validity depends on drawing the boundaries between adjacent syndromes, and between these syndromes and normality, where there are genuine discontinuities either in symptomatology or in etiology. The first stage in defining a syndrome and giving it a provisional definition—which establishes its provisional boundaries—lies in the "five phases" of clinical investigation described by Robins and Guze in 1970. However, this is only the first stage. Ideally, we need to demonstrate either that a "point of rarity" (Sneath 1957) exists between the syndrome in question and other neighboring syndromes or that the boundaries of the syndrome correspond with discontinuities in the relationship between symptomatology and outcome, response to treatment, heritability, or some other validating criterion. Several attempts have been made to do this in the past 30 years, mostly with rather disappointing results.

A number of attempts have been made, by use of discriminant function analysis, to determine whether the symptom patterns of related syndromes merge insensibly into one another or whether a point, or zone, of rarity can be demonstrated between them; in other words, to find out whether mixed forms—"the grays"—are more or less common than typical forms—"the blacks" and "the whites." Two representative data sets are required for this. The first is used to derive a linear discriminant function that provides maximal discrimination between the two syndromes. The scores of the second set of patients on this discriminant function are then plotted out to see whether their distribution is unimodal or bimodal (Figure 1-1).

Gourlay and I used this technique in 1970 to see whether we could demonstrate points of rarity between schizophrenic psychoses and affective psychoses and also between what were then known as endogenous (or psychotic) depressions and reactive (or neurotic) depressions. In both cases we failed (Kendell and Gourlay 1970a, 1970b). Subsequently, Cloninger

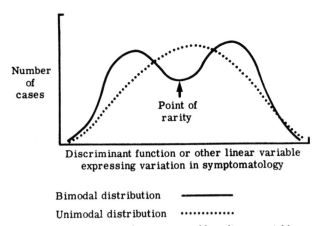

FIGURE 1-1 Variation in symptomatology expressed by a linear variable.
Source. Reprinted from Kendell RE, Brockington IF: "The Identification of Disease Entities and the Relationship Between Schizophrenic and Affective Psychoses." *Br J Psychiatry* 137:324–331, 1980. Used with permission.

and his colleagues in St. Louis, Missouri (Cloninger et al. 1985), used the same method to discriminate between schizophrenia and a mixture of all other psychiatric syndromes. They succeeded, and to my knowledge this is still the only successful demonstration of a point of rarity between psychiatric syndromes.

Brockington and I tried to demonstrate a discontinuity in the relationship between symptomatology and outcome in a mixed population of 127 patients with schizophrenic and affective psychoses for whom we had extensive follow-up information (Kendell and Brockington 1980). This involved plotting the mean scores of these 127 patients on six different indices of outcome against their scores on a discriminant function representing the variation in symptomatology from typical or textbook schizophrenia through schizoaffective states to typical affective psychosis to find out whether the relationship was linear or nonlinear (Figure 1-2).

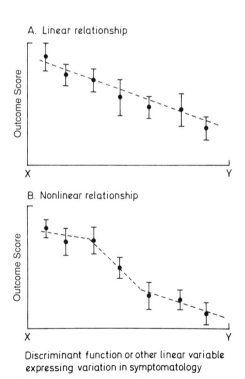

FIGURE 1-2 Relationship between symptomatology and outcome when symtomatology is converted to a linear variable.

Source. Reprinted from Kendell RE, Brockington IF: "The Identification of Disease Entities and the Relationship Between Schizophrenic and Affective Psychoses." *Br J Psychiatry* 137:324–331, 1980. Used with permission.

Possibly because our numbers were too small and our confidence limits were therefore very wide, we were unable to demonstrate any discontinuity.

Recently, Kendler and Gardner (1998) used the same technique to find out whether a valid boundary could be demonstrated between major depression, as defined in DSM-IV, and lesser degrees of depression. Their case material consisted of 2,000 female twins for whom they had extensive follow-up information, and they examined the relationship between depressive symptomatology and both the risk of further depressive episodes in the probands and the risk of major depression in their cotwins. They failed to find any evidence of discontinuity in either relationship and were forced to conclude that "major depression . . . may be a diagnostic convention imposed on a continuum of depressive symptoms of varying severity and duration" (p. 172).

Clearly these half-dozen studies do not justify any firm conclusions. It is entirely possible that further analyses of more extensive data from large, representative populations will demonstrate replicable points of rarity between related syndromes or stable discontinuities in the relationship between symptomatology and outcome, treatment response, or heritability. We have to accept, though, that at present we have little evidence that the boundaries we have drawn between most of the 200 recognized syndromes are based on natural boundaries. We do not know, in other words, whether we are "carving nature at the joints" or even whether there are any "joints," or discontinuities, to be found.

A more popular and probably more powerful way of establishing the validity of clinical syndromes is to elucidate their etiology. There are, of course, other important reasons for exploring etiology. Understanding of underlying mechanisms often leads to more effective therapies and sometimes to a means of preventing a disorder from developing at all. This is why a high proportion of all research into mental disorders is concerned, directly or indirectly, with their etiology, and major etiological discoveries often involve the incidental benefit of validating the clinical syndrome. The demonstrations at various stages in the past 100 years that general paralysis of the insane (GPI) was associated with spirochaetal infection of the brain, that Alzheimer's disease had a specific histopathology, that Down syndrome was accompanied by trisomy of chromosome 21, that Renpenning syndrome was associated with a trinucleotide repeat on the X chromosome, and that Huntington's chorea was associated with an abnormal gene on chromosome 4 all established the validity of the associated clinical syndrome. Indeed, they did more than that. In each case the association between the clinical syndrome and the underlying abnormality was so strong that the abnormality replaced the clinical syndrome as the "defining characteristic" of the disease. Moreover, each of these etiological discoveries involved the demonstration of a discontinuity. Few things are more clearly discontinuous than an abnormal gene or an additional chromosome present only in members of a well-defined clinical category.

These examples are all well known because they are rare. As we are all painfully aware, mental disorders are unique in contemporary medicine because most of them are still defined by their clinical syndromes. Originally, of course, all diseases were defined in this way, but in other branches of medicine the great majority are now defined at some more fundamental level. Only dermatology and neurology still share with psychiatry the dubious distinction of continuing to define a significant proportion of their disorders by their syndromes.

One of the reasons, and perhaps the most important reason, why a predominantly syndrome-based classification like that of psychiatry should be as valid as possible is that accurate delineation of clinical syndromes makes it easier to elucidate their etiology. Noguchi would have found it much harder to demonstrate the syphilitic origin of GPI if clinicians had not already been able to discriminate fairly accurately between GPI and other dementias, and Gusella and his colleagues might have failed to identify the abnormal gene on chromosome 4 if Huntington's disease had not been well discriminated from other dementias and choreas. Sometimes, however, the sequence of discovery is reversed. In the case of phenylketonuria, it was Fölling's identification of phenylpyruvic acid in the urine of some children with mental handicaps that made it possible to delineate the associated clinical syndrome (fair hair and skin, short stature, hyperactivity, eczema, and convulsions).

PROSPECTS FOR A BETTER TAXONOMY

Now that we have achieved adequate reliability, the most important weakness of taxonomies of mental disorders is the uncertain validity of the majority of their categories. For this reason future classifications are unlikely to be regarded as significantly better unless they possess demonstrably higher validity. This implies that the prospects for a better taxonomy of mental disorders largely depend on the prospects of our producing or acquiring, within the next decade or two, substantially better evidence than we have at present of the validity of some of the major categories of mental disorder.

This might be achieved by a more meticulous and determined analysis of clinical and epidemiological data. Discriminant function analysis of clinical ratings (derived by structured interviewing methods) from large, representative populations and sustained attempts—such as that by Kendler and Gardner (1998)—to demonstrate discontinuities in the relationship between symptomatology and response to treatment, outcome, or heritability might provide the evidence that our operational definitions do indeed put the boundaries in the appropriate places. Alternatively, such research might provide cogent evidence that a boundary—either between two neighboring syndromes or between a clinical syndrome and normality—should be moved or abolished.

I hope that more investigations of this kind will be carried out in the next decade than in the past. Even so, they are not likely to solve many of our outstanding problems. It is important to appreciate that failures to demonstrate the presence of a valid boundary, like that experienced by Kendler and Gardner, never prove that there is no boundary to be found. It is always possible that a different selection of clinical ratings or a different validating criterion to plot against symptomatology might reveal a critical discontinuity.

In the absence of clear evidence of points of rarity and discontinuities, the possibility of representing variation in symptomatology by dimensions rather than by categories needs to be considered. The idea is not new. Wittenborn and colleagues (1953) developed an elaborate nine-dimensional representation of the phenomena of psychotic illness 50 years ago, and others have subsequently developed and advocated dimensional models to portray the symptomatology of depressive (Kendell 1968) and chronic schizophrenic (Liddle 1987) illnesses and the whole field of psychopathology (Eysenck 1970). Dimensional representation solves at a stroke all the problems associated with boundaries and comorbidity and may also be a powerful means of predicting outcome. Even so, there is no foreseeable prospect that any formal national or international classification will adopt a dimensional format, except possibly for personality disorders. The rest of medicine is too firmly committed to categories, and in any case dimensions are better suited to the portrayal of variation in populations than to day-to-day decisions about the treatment of individuals. This does not mean, however, that dimensional systems may not have an important role for research purposes or as an experimental alternative to an established typology. Indeed, they should be more widely used than they are.

ETIOLOGICAL UNDERSTANDING

The strongest and most convincing evidence for the validity, or lack of validity, of our present taxonomies is likely to come from etiological research, and substantial resources and the skills of many multidisciplinary research teams are going to be devoted to this quest in the next 20 years, particularly into the genetic basis of mental disorders and functional magnetic resonance imaging studies of these disorders. The critical question therefore is, how likely is this research to generate findings that will either validate several of the important categories in our existing taxonomies or provide new and more valid categories to replace them?

In the long run it is bound to do so. The only reason most mental disorders are still defined by their clinical syndromes is that the human brain is an infinitely more complex machine with a much wider range of functions than the heart, the kidney, or the liver. It is also much more complex than the brains of other mammals. We therefore have more difficulty understanding its disorders. In time we undoubtedly will. However, it may be a long time before we understand some of its more sophisticated functions, such as storing memories (but only important ones) and generating and interpreting speech, and an even longer time before we understand the disorders of these remarkable abilities.

Over the next 20 years or so we will undoubtedly learn a great deal about the genetic basis of most mental disorders. Many susceptibility genes will be identified and their protein products identified and sequenced. Functional magnetic resonance imaging and other brain-scanning technologies will provide detailed information about the areas of the brain involved in psychological functions such as vision, hearing, memory, and speech and about which areas are either underactive or overactive in people with particular mental disorders. We can be confident, too, that epidemiology will provide important new information about environmental risk factors and that investigation of the modes of action of psychotropic drugs, and new fields of research and new technologies that at present we have not even begun to dream of, will also provide new information and new lines of inquiry.

In 20 years' time we will have a considerably broader and deeper understanding of the etiology and the pathophysiology of several mental disorders than we do at present. I think it is doubtful, however, whether this new information and understanding will validate many of our existing categories or enable us to replace them with valid new categories.

We already have strong evidence that genetic factors make a major contribution to a wide range of mental disorders. Unfortunately for nosologists, it seems increasingly likely that in most situations this genetically determined susceptibility will prove to depend on many different genes acting and interacting in several different ways, and that each on its own will be responsible for only a modest increase in risk. It seems likely, too, that some of these genes contribute to several different disorders: to the broad territory of anxiety and depression, for example, or to both schizophrenic and affective psychoses. Our more limited understanding of the environmental determinants of mental disorders suggests that these too are rarely specific to a single disorder or group of obviously related disorders and that they interact with genetically determined susceptibilities in many different ways and at different stages of development.

An etiological framework of this kind does not lend itself to a categorical classification of disorders, unless the complex interactions of genetic and environmental factors produce a single well-defined pathology that underlies and accounts for the clinical syndrome. It may be, for example, that in Alzheimer's disease, although a variety of complex interactions among genetically determined variations in neuronal metabolism and environmental factors (such as head injury and duration of education) contribute to the formation of amyloid plaques, it is those plaques that lead to neuronal death and the progressive cognitive decline of the illness. If this proves to be so, amyloid plaques will be confirmed as the defining characteristic of the condition. Only time will tell whether schizophrenia, bipolar disorder, and obsessional disorder will eventually prove to have comparable well-defined pathologies underlying and accounting for their clinical manifestations. I doubt, however, whether we will know the answers to these questions within the next 10 or even the next 20 years.

DSM-V

The American Psychiatric Association (APA) has already decided to produce a new, fifth edition of its *Diagnostic and Statistical Manual of Mental Disorders* (DSM-V), and this will probably come into use some time between 2007 and 2010. We can be sure that much time and energy and a great deal of expertise will be devoted to this new taxonomy. Comprehensive literature reviews will be carried out, groups of experts will be appointed to revise every section and to reconsider the wording of every operational definition, and field trials of various kinds will be mounted. At the end of the day it is likely that DSM-V will differ from DSM-IV in many comparatively minor ways and that most of these changes will be seen as improvements by most American experts and researchers studying a particular group of disorders. It is less likely that the changes will be regarded as improvements by the much larger population of ordinary clinicians who will probably find themselves committed to using this new classification and glossary by their employers or reimbursers. Changes in classifications or definitions are always disruptive and always involve losses as well as gains. Ordinary clinicians are liable to be confused or irritated by changes they see no need for or may simply ignore them. Academics and research workers who understand the reasons for the changes may be more welcoming, but even they have to cope with the fact that, because the new categories and definitions are subtly different from those in use for the past decade, they will be uncertain whether the information in the literature of the past decade about prevalence, treatment response, and outcome can still be relied on. There is a risk, too, as Kendler (1990) pointed out, that frequent changes of definition based on nothing more substantial than a swing in expert opinion may undermine the credibility of psychiatric nosology.

I am not suggesting that the APA was ill advised to commit itself at this stage to producing a new edition of the DSM; merely that DSM-V is likely to represent a fairly modest advance on DSM-IV and that the changeover from IV to V will involve losses as well as gains. It is not unreasonable to produce a new edition after what is likely to be an interval of more than 12 years. Indeed, between 1948 and 1992 WHO produced five revisions of the ICD, roughly one every decade. The decision to produce a new manual will stimulate research that might not otherwise have been done and further discussion of fundamental issues such as how best to define "mental disorder." It also provides an opportunity to update the classification of groups of disorders, such as the dementias, in which there have been genuine advances and increasing understanding of etiology in the past decade. It is important, however, that changes be as limited as possible overall and firmly evidence based.

At present, WHO has no plans to produce a new revision of the ICD, but this is primarily for financial reasons. The APA makes a handsome profit on each new edition of its DSM, but it is a costly undertaking for WHO to produce a new revision of the ICD. Each revision involves a series of expensive international meetings, many of them with simultaneous translation into several different languages, and the finished product has to be formally approved by nearly 200 different countries and then translated into the eight official languages of the United Nations. Indeed, the main reason for introducing an alphanumeric format in ICD-10 was to create spare capacity in the taxonomy and thereby give it a longer working life.

As I understand it, American psychiatrists are currently expected, both by the bodies that fund health care and by the editors of North American journals, to use the categories and definitions of DSM-IV, and this is likely to be so for DSM-V as well. Although there are understandable reasons for this, and indeed some advantages, conformity to a single approved taxonomy and a single set of operational definitions also discourages innovation. Clinical researchers should not merely be allowed but should be positively encouraged to use radically new operational definitions and syndromal groupings, or dimensional representations, if they see good reasons for doing so, and then to present the relationships they are concerned with as two parallel sets of analyses, one using conventional definitions like those of the current DSM or ICD and the other using their own novel definition in order to allow the two to be compared. The core of our current dilemma is that we will never be certain where to draw the boundary between one syndrome and the next until we understand the underlying mechanisms, and we will have difficulty identifying these mechanisms unless we have the clinical boundaries in the right places first. In this situation, as Strauss and Gift (1977) pointed out in the early days of operational definitions, there are advantages in having more than one string to one's bow.

REFERENCES

American Psychiatric Association: Diagnostic and Statistical Manual of Mental Disorders, 2nd Edition. Washington, DC, American Psychiatric Association, 1968

American Psychiatric Association: Diagnostic and Statistical Manual of Mental Disorders, 3rd Edition. Washington, DC, American Psychiatric Association, 1980

American Psychiatric Association: Diagnostic and Statistical Manual of Mental Disorders, 3rd Edition, Revised. Washington, DC, American Psychiatric Association, 1987

American Psychiatric Association: Diagnostic and Statistical Manual of Mental Disorders, 4th Edition. Washington, DC, American Psychiatric Association, 1994

Cloninger CR, Martin RL, Guze SB, et al: Diagnosis and prognosis in psychiatry. Arch Gen Psychiatry 42:15–25, 1985

Dunnell K and Cartwright A: Medicine Takers, Prescribers and Hoarders. London, England, Routledge & Kegan Paul, 1972

Eysenck HJ: A dimensional system of psychodiagnostics, in New Approaches to Personality Classification. Edited by Mahrer AR. New York, Columbia University Press, 1970, pp 169–207

Kendell RE: The Classification of Depressive Illnesses (Maudsley Monograph No 18). London, England, Oxford University Press, 1968

Kendell RE: The concept of disease and its implications for psychiatry. Br J Psychiatry 127:305–315, 1975

Kendell RE: What are mental disorders? in Issues in Psychiatric Classification: Science, Practice and Social Policy. Edited by Freedman AM, Brotman R, Silverman I, et al. New York, Human Sciences Press, 1986, pp 23–45

Kendell RE, Brockington IF: The identification of disease entities and the relationship between schizophrenic and affective psychoses. Br J Psychiatry 137:324–331, 1980

Kendell RE, Gourlay J: The clinical distinction between psychotic and neurotic depression. Br J Psychiatry 117:257–260, 1970a

Kendell RE, Gourlay J: The clinical distinction between the affective psychoses and schizophrenia. Br J Psychiatry 117:261–266, 1970b

Kendler KS: Towards a scientific nosology. Arch Gen Psychiatry 47:969–973, 1990

Kendler KS: Setting boundaries for psychiatric disorders. Am J Psychiatry 156:1845–1848, 1999

Kendler KS, Gardner CO: Boundaries of major depression: an evaluation of DSM-IV criteria. Am J Psychiatry 155:172–177, 1998

Kessler RC, McGonagle KA, Zhao S, et al: Lifetime and 12-month prevalence of DSM-III-R psychiatric disorders in the United States: results from the National Comorbidity Survey. Arch Gen Psychiatry 51:8–19, 1994

Liddle PF: The symptoms of chronic schizophrenia: a re-examination of the positive–negative dichotomy. Br J Psychiatry 151:145–151, 1987

Robins E, Guze SB: Establishment of diagnostic validity in psychiatric illness: its application to schizophrenia. Am J Psychiatry 126:983–987, 1970

Robins LN, Regier DA: Psychiatric Disorders in America. New York, Free Press, 1991

Sneath PHA: Some thoughts on bacterial classification. J Gen Microbiol 17:184–200, 1957

Spitzer RL, Wakefield JC: DSM-IV diagnostic criterion for clinical significance: does it help solve the false positive problem? Am J Psychiatry 156:1856–1864, 1999

Strauss JS, Gift TE: Choosing an approach for diagnosing schizophrenia. Arch Gen Psychiatry 34:1248–1253, 1977

Wadsworth MEJ, Blaney R, Butterfield WJH: Health and Sickness: The Choice of Treatment. London, England, Tavistock Press, 1971

Wakefield JC: The concept of mental disorder: on the boundary between biological facts and social values. Am Psychol 47:373–388, 1992

Wittenborn JR, Holzberg JD, Simon B: Symptom correlates for descriptive diagnosis. Genetic Psychology Monographs 47:237–301, 1953

World Health Organization: International Classification of Impairments, Disabilities, and Handicaps. Geneva, Switzerland, World Health Organization, 1980

World Health Organization: The ICD-10 Classification of Mental and Behavioural Disorders: Clinical Descriptions and Diagnostic Guidelines. Geneva, Switzerland, World Health Organization, 1992

2

Defining Clinically Significant Psychopathology With Epidemiologic Data

Darrel A. Regier, M.D., M.P.H.
William E. Narrow, M.D., M.P.H.

The development of both psychiatric epidemiology and the underlying conceptual framework of psychiatric nosology is currently at an interesting crossroads. This historical period comes after two major national epidemiological surveys with multiple international replications over the past 20 years and just at the start of serious consideration for a DSM-IV (American Psychiatric Association 1994) revision.

The Epidemiologic Catchment Area (ECA) program (Robins and Regier 1991; Regier et al. 1984) and the third edition of the *Diagnostic and Statistical Manual of Mental Disorders* (DSM-III; American Psychiatric Association 1980) were introduced simultaneously in 1980, during which time the close working relationship between Robert Spitzer and Lee Robins benefited the development of the Diagnostic Interview Schedule (Robins et al. 1981) used in the ECA program. The ECA program was a five-site study of approximately 20,000 adults ages 18 years and older involving a 1-year prospective design that included both community and institutionalized populations. It was able to provide extensive information on the prevalence of mental disorders defined by the explicit criteria of DSM-III that were embedded in the Diagnostic Interview Schedule. In addition, it provided significant details on sociodemographic correlates or risk factors and extensive information on a full range of health and human services used by

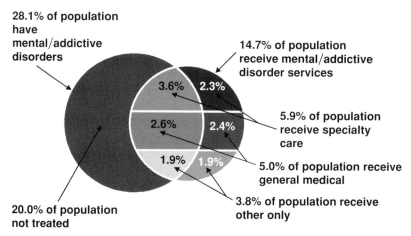

28.1% of population have mental/addictive disorders

14.7% of population receive mental/addictive disorder services

5.9% of population receive specialty care

5.0% of population receive general medical

3.8% of population receive other only

20.0% of population not treated

FIGURE 2-1   Annual prevalence of mental/addictive disorders and services.

subjects to help with these conditions. Figure 2-1 summarizes the 1-year mental and addictive disorder prevalence findings and the 1-year mental and addictive disorder treatment service use of subjects in the ECA program (Regier et al. 1993).

A decade later, the National Comorbidity Survey (NCS; Kessler et al. 1994) was supported by the National Institute of Mental Health (NIMH) to replicate certain aspects of the ECA program and to obtain more detailed information on the timing and sequence of onset and remission of specific mental and addictive disorders. To focus on age groups most likely to have comorbid mental and addictive disorders, a younger age group of approximately 8,000 people ages 15–54 years was surveyed from a national probability sample of community residents only. DSM-III-R (American Psychiatric Association 1987) criteria were used for the University of Michigan version of the Composite International Diagnostic Interview (UM-CIDI; Robins et al. 1988; Wittchen and Kessler 1994), which was the case identification or diagnostic instrument used in the NCS. Although most of the diagnostic criteria were relatively similar between DSM-III and DSM-III-R, there were also some notable exceptions, such as social phobia, which was given additional gateways of entry by the expanded diagnostic criteria in DSM-III-R. Because there were differences in population age groups, instrument design, the single-wave survey design of the NCS, and prevalence rates of some specific disorders, it was somewhat surprising to find relatively similar overall 1-year prevalence rates (Table 2-1).

In an earlier publication (Regier et al. 1998), prevalence discrepancies between the ECA program and the NCS were analyzed and found to be largely attributable to differences in age, urban versus rural residence,

TABLE 2-1   12-month prevalence of mental disorders, ages 18–54

Disorder	NCS data	ECA data
Any mood disorder	11.1	10.4
Major depressive episode	10.1	6.5
Manic episode	1.3	1.2
Dysthymia	2.5	5.7[a]
Any anxiety disorder	18.7	13.3
Panic disorder	2.2	1.6
Agoraphobia	3.7	5.0
Social phobia	7.4	2.0
Simple phobia	8.6	8.5
Any phobia	14.7	11.4
Generalized anxiety disorder	3.4	—
Obsessive-compulsive disorder	—	2.3
Any substance use disorder	11.5	11.7
Alcohol abuse or dependence	9.9	9.1
Drug abuse or dependence	3.6	4.0
Schizophrenia/nonaffective psychosis	0.2	1.3
Any mental or substance use disorder	30.2	29.6

[a]Lifetime rate.
ECA = Epidemiologic Catchment Area; NCS = National Comorbidity Survey.

instrument structure, and diagnostic criteria. When these variables were controlled, the differences between the two surveys could be narrowed. Especially noteworthy are the prevalence rate changes that occurred within the NCS when DSM-III criteria were applied to the NCS data (Table 2-2), particularly among the anxiety disorders, for which rates were more than halved from 15.6% to 7.2%. The marked increase in rates from DSM-III to

TABLE 2-2   National Comorbidity Survey prevalence with DSM-III and DSM-III-R: anxiety disorders

Disorder	DSM-III	DSM-III-R
Social phobia	3.2	8.1
Simple phobia	3.4	8.5
Agoraphobia	1.9	3.1
Any phobia	6.6	14.9
Panic disorder	1.4	2.1
Any anxiety disorder	7.2	15.6
Any mental or substance use disorder	22.8	28.6

Note. Because of the different sample definitions, the DSM-III-R National Comorbidity Survey prevalence rates do not match those in other tables (see Regier et al. 1998).

DSM-III-R was influenced primarily by rates of social phobia and simple phobia, which both increased from approximately 3% to approximately 8%—primarily because of the expanded entry criteria. Also, Table 2-2 shows that the total disorder rate for any diagnosis in the NCS increased from 22.8% under DSM-III to 28.6% under DSM-III-R.

More recently, we have focused attention on the implications of DSM-IV, which introduced a "clinical significance" criterion to previous diagnostic criteria that had emerged from earlier DSM and International Classification of Diseases (ICD) revisions (American Psychiatric Association 1994; Frances 1998; Narrow et al., in press). This DSM-IV criterion requires clinically significant (or marked) distress or significant interference with social, occupational, or other areas of functioning. We reanalyzed both the ECA program and the NCS by using new scoring algorithms, which operationalize clinical significance criteria (Narrow et al., in press). These analyses are based on data from ECA and NCS probes that were placed at either the symptom or the syndrome level of scoring. In the ECA program, the clinical significance questions were as follows: Did you tell a doctor about (symptom[s])?; Did you tell any other professional about (symptom[s])?; Did you take medicine for (symptom[s]) more than once?; Did (symptom[s]) interfere with your life or activities a lot? The NCS included the following clinical significance questions: Did you ever tell a doctor other than a psychiatrist about (symptom[s])?; Did you ever see a mental health specialist about your (symptom[s])?; Did you ever see any other professional about (symptom[s])?; Did you ever take medication more than once because of (symptom[s])?; How much did your (symptom[s]) ever interfere with your life or activities—a lot, some, a little, or not at all? Despite their limitations, these questions are our best approximation of the DSM-IV clinical significance requirement through use of currently available data.

TABLE 2-3   National Comorbidity Survey prevalence before and after clinical significance criteria: anxiety disorders

Disorder	Before clinical significance: DSM-III-R	After clinical significance: DSM-IV
Social phobia	7.4	3.7
Simple phobia	8.6	4.4
Agoraphobia	3.7	2.2
Any phobia	14.7	8.0
Panic disorder	2.2	1.7
Generalized anxiety disorder	3.4	2.8
Posttraumatic stress disorder	3.6	3.6
Any anxiety disorder	18.7	12.1

Source. Data from Narrow et al., in press.

TABLE 2-4 National Comorbidity Survey prevalence before and after clinical significance criteria: mood disorders

Disorder	Before clinical significance: DSM-III-R	After clinical significance: DSM-IV
Major depressive episode	10.1	6.4
Unipolar major depressive disorder	8.9	5.4
Dysthymia	2.5	1.8
Bipolar I disorder	1.3	1.3
Bipolar II disorder	—	0.2
Any mood disorder	11.1	7.5

Source. Data from Narrow et al., in press.

For major depression in the ECA program and most disorders in the NCS, the probes were assessed at the syndrome level instead of at the symptom level. This means that clinical significance questions were asked about a group of positive symptoms, and as a result, the syndrome could be clinically significant or not clinically significant. For our analysis, we considered a positive response to any one of the clinical significance questions (for the life interference question in the NCS, "a lot") to be indicative of a clinically significant syndrome. When these criteria were applied to the NCS anxiety disorders (Table 2-3), there was a significant drop in prevalence rates of the phobias from approximately 15% to 8%. Any anxiety disorder dropped from approximately 19% to 12%. Prevalence rates of mood disorders decreased from 11% to 7.5% (Table 2-4). Overall, mental and substance use disorders decreased from 30.2% to 20.6%—approximately a 30% drop (Table 2-5).

For the ECA anxiety disorders, the clinical significance questions were asked at the symptom level only, with no probes at the syndrome level. A symptom could not be coded as present by the ECA interviewer unless one of the clinical significance questions was positive. As a result, the ECA rates for anxiety disorders are automatically clinically significant rates.

TABLE 2-5 National Comorbidity Survey prevalence before and after clinical significance criteria: substance use disorders and all disorders

Disorder	Before clinical significance: DSM-III-R	After clinical significance: DSM-IV
Any mental disorder	23.4	15.4
Any substance use disorder	11.5	7.6
Any mental or substance use disorder	30.2	20.6

Source. Data from Narrow et al., in press.

TABLE 2-6   Epidemiologic Catchment Area prevalence before and after clinical significance criteria: mood disorders, ages 18+

Disorder	Before clinical significance: DSM-III-R	After clinical significance: DSM-IV
Major depressive episode	5.8	4.5
Unipolar major depressive disorder	4.9	4.0
Dysthymia	5.5[a]	1.7[b]
Bipolar I disorder	0.9	0.5
Bipolar II disorder	0.4	0.2
Any mood disorder	9.5	5.1

[a]Lifetime rate. [b]1-year rate.
Source. Data from Narrow et al., in press.

It is noteworthy that the NCS rate for any anxiety disorder, which used syndrome-level probes, actually dropped below that of the ECA rate. For major depression in the ECA program, clinical significance questions were asked at the syndrome level but were not used in previously published analyses. Hence, when the criteria are applied, there is a drop in overall prevalence rates as shown in Table 2-6. Overall, ECA prevalence rates for any mental disorder dropped to approximately 17% and the rate for any mental or addictive disorder dropped from 28.0% to 22.5% (Table 2-7).

To assess the correlates of these new rates in terms of service use and other available indicators of functional impairment and distress, additional analyses were performed with both the ECA and NCS clinically significant disorders. In the first of these, we compared the rates of service use for the clinically significant and nonclinically significant anxiety disorders and unipolar major depression (Table 2-8). As can be seen in both the ECA program and the NCS, there are large differences in the proportions when mental health services are used in all sectors.

Validity indicators that were common between the ECA program and the NCS included full-time work or school attendance, lifetime suicidal

TABLE 2-7   Epidemiologic Catchment Area prevalence before and after clinical significance criteria: substance use disorders and all disorders

Disorder	Before clinical significance: DSM-III-R	After clinical significance: DSM-IV
Any mental disorder	22.0	17.2
Any substance use disorder	9.3	7.7
Any mental or substance use disorder	28.0	22.5

Source. Data from Narrow et al., in press.

ideation, and lifetime suicide attempts (Table 2-9). The suicide indicators were significantly higher for the clinically significant anxiety disorders and major depression. The differences in proportions in full-time work or school were less dramatic. The reasons for this latter finding,

TABLE 2-8   Clinical significance and service use: any anxiety disorder and unipolar major depression

| | Percentage with service use | | | |
| | ECA | | NCS | |
	−CS	+CS	−CS	+CS
Any anxiety disorder				
Specialty	—	16.3	4.0	21.5***
General medical	—	14.8	2.0	13.6***
Health systems[a]	—	27.4	5.6	28.5***
Any service use	—	35.4	9.0	34.7***
Unipolar major depressive disorder				
Specialty	11.9	34.3***	3.5	34.1***
General medical	7.0	30.0***	4.5	17.5***
Health systems[a]	17.9	53.7***	7.5	42.4***
Any service use	30.4	62.9***	9.3	48.6***

[a]Health systems refer to any specialty or general medical service use.
*** $P < 0.001$.
CS = clinical significance; ECA = Epidemiologic Catchment Area; NCS = National Comorbidity Survey.
Source. Data from Narrow et al., in press.

TABLE 2-9   Validity indicators: any anxiety disorder and unipolar major depressive disorder

| | Percentage with indicator | | | |
| | ECA | | NCS | |
	−CS	+CS	−CS	+CS
Any anxiety disorder				
Full-time work or school	—	56.5	58.6	51.0*
Suicidal ideation	—	33.3	27.2	47.4***
Suicide attempt	—	12.4	6.5	19.5***
Unipolar major depressive disorder				
Full-time work or school	62.7	54.2	49.9	56.8
Suicidal ideation	29.0	58.5***	35.7	57.8***
Suicide attempt	6.5	21.2***	7.3	21.1***

*** $P < 0.001$; ** $P < 0.01$; * $P < 0.05$.
CS = clinical significance; ECA = Epidemiologic Catchment Area; NCS = National Comorbidity Survey.
Source. Data from Narrow et al., in press.

TABLE 2-10   Best estimate prevalence rates, ages 18 and older

Any mental disorder	14.9
Any substance use disorder	6.0
Any mental or substance use disorder	18.5

Source. Data from Narrow et al., in press.

whether methodological or indicative of the clinical nature of these disorders, should be studied further.

Combining the most conservative estimates from both the ECA program and NCS resulted in a composite "best-estimate" annual prevalence of 15% for any mental disorder, 6% for any substance use disorder, and a total of approximately 18.5% for any mental or substance use disorder (Table 2-10). We were able to compare our findings with preliminary data from the Australian National Survey (G. Andrews, personal communication, November 1998). In this survey, DSM-IV clinical significance criteria were operationalized, whereas the ICD-10 (World Health Organization [WHO] 1992) criteria were left without such restrictions. In these preliminary findings, the overall DSM-IV rate, without exclusions, was approximately 17% compared with an ICD-10 rate of 23% (Table 2-11). However, Andrews estimates that the inclusion of cognitive impairment, personality disorders, somatization, and schizophrenia would increase the DSM-IV rate to approximately 20%.

If one were to summarize the overall prevalence rate relationships associated with DSM-III, DSM-III-R, and DSM-IV criteria, it would appear that the lowest or most conservative rates are obtained by DSM-IV, followed by DSM-III, with DSM-III-R having the highest rates. There also appears to be an inverse relationship between the annual disorder

TABLE 2-11   Australian national mental health survey: 1-year DSM-IV and ICD-10 prevalence rates

Disorders	DSM-IV	ICD-10
Any anxiety disorder	8.1	10.9
Any mood disorder	6.6	7.2
Any mental or addictive disorder	17.1	23.3

Source. Data from G. Andrews, personal communication, November 1998 and Andrews G: "Meeting the Unmet Need With Disease Management," in *Unmet Need in Psychiatry: Problems, Resources, Responses.* Edited by Andrews G, Henderson S. Cambridge, United Kingdom, Cambridge University Press, 2000, pp. 11–36.

prevalence rates and the proportion of those with disorders receiving treatment, that is, the clinically significant DSM-IV–defined disorders, which have the lowest rates, are associated with the highest level of service use.

Despite the reassurance that clinically significant disorders may be closer approximations of need for care, diagnosis by itself is not a sufficient indicator of treatment need. Many subthreshold anxiety and mood disorders also have been shown to have significant associated impairment (Horwath et al. 1994; Judd et al. 1997; Olfson et al. 1996). In a primary care study that NIMH conducted in the late 1970s at the Marshfield Clinic in Wisconsin, we were able to demonstrate that the Global Assessment Scale (GAS), now referred to as the Global Assessment of Functioning Scale (GAF) in DSM, was a much more efficient predictor of service use than Research Diagnostic Criteria (RDC) criteria or a score on the General Health Questionnaire symptom scale (Regier et al. 1985). Hence, the need for additional measures of functional impairment has become obvious over the past 25 years. The SF-36 and SF-12 were used for measuring functional impairment in the recent Dutch (Bijl et al. 1998) and Australian (Henderson et al. 2000) national surveys. In addition, both of these surveys also assessed the number of days in the past month in which the person was unable to work or carry out his or her usual activities for health reasons, which may become a better empirical basis for assessing Disability Adjusted Life Years in the WHO World Bank Global Burden of Disease paradigm (Murray and Lopez 1996). The WHO Disability Assessment Scale (WHO-DAS) will provide another measure of disability across the full range of physical and mental disorders, of potential use for judging treatment need. In addition to disability, symptom scales such as the Hamilton depression and anxiety scales have become standard measures for assessing severity and response to treatment in clinical trials. For example, it is clearly possible to meet all criteria for major depressive disorder, but with symptom severity low enough that the disorder would generally not be seen as requiring treatment.

In his upcoming epidemiological surveys in the United States and in several countries around the world, Ronald Kessler has indicated an interest in using some combination of disability and symptom measures that would be specific for each disorder. Although this approach is a logical extension of the experience that has been gained by the field of epidemiology over the past 20 years, the battery of instruments planned for these studies has not yet become available. Where does this leave us as we attempt to draw on research experience to recommend improvements in future diagnostic criteria that will be both more valid and more indicative of treatment need?

1. We need to use both epidemiological and clinical studies to test the hypotheses that the existing diagnostic criteria are valid indicators of psychopathology and treatment need. Available evidence indicates that many people who meet diagnostic criteria for disorders have neither functional impairment nor a perceived need for treatment. Hence, some adjustments in the criteria—particularly those that would operationalize clinical significance seem appropriate.
2. It may be possible to develop some better staging of disorders that would have implications for treatment need as has been done in the field of cancer diagnosis and treatment. Such staging could be done with a combination of both symptom and impairment criteria.
3. The need to improve our definition of psychopathology has significant scientific implications as we attempt to define phenotypes for genetic studies. In general, the criteria of Robins and Guze for psychopathology validity require substantial refinements in available diagnostic systems.
4. Definitions of disorders will never fully encompass the concept of treatment need because functional impairment associated with subsyndromal disorders will continue to require clinical attention. For example, few researchers would debate the treatment need of an acutely suicidal person who did not quite meet full diagnostic criteria for major depressive disorder or any other mental disorder. However, scientific skepticism remains about whether the prevalence rates being generated by existing criteria are accurate reflections of the level of true psychopathology in the population.

The policy implications of epidemiologic survey research continue to resonate as journalists and policymakers respond to the recent Surgeon General's report on mental health (U.S. Department of Health and Human Services 1999), which noted that approximately one-fifth of the population meets criteria for a mental disorder alone in 1 year, increasing to approximately 28%–30% when addictive disorders are added. In addition, mental health systems in both public and private areas continue to compete for shrinking health care dollars. The "best estimate" prevalence of 18.5% for mental and addictive disorders that emerged from our recent analysis represents a decrease from the previous ECA estimate of 28.1% of almost 19 million adults age 18 years and older. These lower numbers are likely to represent a group in greater need of services, but the remaining numbers remain overwhelming for planning purposes (Narrow et al., in press).

Thus, a major goal of the next generation of psychiatric epidemiology will be to establish a more precise and clinically relevant baseline than was accomplished by the ECA program and the NCS. Full advantage should be taken of advances in the operationalization of disability constructs and symptom scales and their translation into survey instruments. Longitudinal designs are needed to determine course of illness and changes in functional levels over time—starting with childhood-onset disorders (Narrow et al., in press).

Until we are able to identify pathognomonic biological markers, such as functional imaging patterns complemented by genetic traits, we will remain dependent on observational criteria of syndromes, clinical course, impairment levels, treatment response, and familial aggregation to inform our definitions of psychopathology and need for treatment. New hypotheses will be embedded in the DSM-V to replace those that have proven inadequate in previous iterations to separate normal variations from pathological states requiring treatment interventions.

REFERENCES

American Psychiatric Association: Diagnostic and Statistical Manual of Mental Disorders, 3rd Edition. Washington, DC, American Psychiatric Association, 1980

American Psychiatric Association: Diagnostic and Statistical Manual of Mental Disorders, 3rd Edition, Revised. Washington, DC, American Psychiatric Association, 1987

American Psychiatric Association: Diagnostic and Statistical Manual of Mental Disorders, 4th Edition. Washington, DC, American Psychiatric Association, 1994

Bijl RV, van Zessen G, Ravelli A, et al: The Netherlands Mental Health Survey and Incidence Study (NEMESIS): objectives and design. Soc Psychiatry Psychiatr Epidemiol 33:581–586, 1998

Frances A: Problems in defining clinical significance in epidemiological studies. Arch Gen Psychiatry 55:119, 1998

Henderson S, Andrews G, Hall W: Australia's mental health: an overview of the general population survey. Aust N Z J Psychiatry 34:197–205, 2000

Horwath E, Johnson J, Klerman GL, et al: What are the public health implications of subclinical depressive symptoms? Psychiatr Q 65:323–337, 1994

Judd LL, Akiskal HS, Paulus MP: The role and clinical significance of subsyndromal depressive symptoms (SSD) in unipolar major depressive disorder. J Affect Disord 45:5–17, 1997

Kessler RC, McGonagle KA, Zhao S, et al: Lifetime and 12-month prevalence of DSM-III-R psychiatric disorders in the United States: results from the National Comorbidity Survey. Arch Gen Psychiatry 51:8–19, 1994

Murray CJL, Lopez AD (eds): The Global Burden of Disease. Boston, MA, Harvard School of Public Health, 1996

Narrow WE, Rae DS, Robins LN, et al: Revised prevalence estimates of mental disorders in the U.S.: using a clinical significance criterion to reconcile two surveys' estimates. Arch Gen Psychiatry (in press)

Olfson M, Broadhead WE, Weissman MM, et al: Subthreshold psychiatric symptoms in a primary care group practice. Arch Gen Psychiatry 53:880–886, 1996

Regier DA, Myers JK, Kramer M, et al: The NIMH Epidemiologic Catchment Area program: historical context, major objectives, and study population characteristics. Arch Gen Psychiatry 41:34–941, 1984

Regier DA, Burke JDJ, Manderscheid RW, et al: The chronically mentally ill in primary care. Psychol Med 15:265–273, 1985

Regier DA, Narrow WE, Rae DS, et al: The de facto US mental and addictive disorders service system: Epidemiologic Catchment Area prospective 1-year prevalence rates of disorders and services. Arch Gen Psychiatry 50:85–94, 1993

Regier DA, Kaelber CT, Rae DS, et al: Limitations of diagnostic criteria and assessment instruments for mental disorders: implications for research and policy. Arch Gen Psychiatry 55:109–115, 1998

Robins LN, Regier DA (eds): Psychiatric Disorders in America. New York, Free Press, 1991

Robins LN, Helzer JE, Croughan J, et al: National Institute of Mental Health Diagnostic Interview Schedule: its history, characteristics, and validity. Arch Gen Psychiatry 38:381–389, 1981

Robins LN, Wing J, Wittchen HU, et al: The Composite International Diagnostic Interview: an epidemiologic instrument suitable for use in conjunction with different diagnostic systems and in different cultures. Arch Gen Psychiatry 45:1069–1077, 1988

U.S. Department of Health and Human Services: Mental Health: A Report of the Surgeon General. Rockville, MD, U.S. Department of Health and Human Services, Substance Abuse and Mental Health Services Administration, Center for Mental Health Services, National Institutes of Health, National Institute of Mental Health, 1999

Wittchen H-U, Kessler RC: Modifications of the CIDI in the National Comorbidity Survey: The Development of the UM-CIDI. NCS Working Paper #2. Ann Arbor, University of Michigan Press, 1994

World Health Organization: International Classification of Diseases and Health Related Problems, 10th Revision. Geneva, World Health Organization, 1992

3

Why Requiring Clinical Significance Does Not Solve Epidemiology's and DSM's Validity Problem

Response to Regier and Narrow

Jerome C. Wakefield, D.S.W., Ph.D.
Robert L. Spitzer, M.D.

Psychiatric epidemiology has a special role to play in the redefinition of DSM disorders in the twenty-first century. One cannot be really certain about the degree to which clinicians and researchers follow DSM-IV (American Psychiatric Association 1994) diagnostic criteria. But we know that psychiatric epidemiologic studies do apply DSM criteria to community populations as literally as possible. We know this because the diagnoses are computer scored based on answers to questions that are operationalizations of the DSM criteria and that are asked in fully structured clinical interviews by lay interviewers. Psychiatric epidemiology thus provides a unique opportunity for assessing the validity of DSM criteria and for suggesting how criteria fare when applied without implicit adjustments or biases that may be present in other settings.

As we look toward DSM-V and consider revisions in diagnostic criteria, it is important that we recognize that psychiatric epidemiology is in a state of crisis. The source of this crisis lies in the results of the two most ambitious and rigorous studies of mental disorders in community settings ever undertaken, the Epidemiologic Catchment Area (ECA) study (Robins and Regier 1991) and the National Comorbidity Survey (NCS) (Kessler et al. 1994). The problem is, first, that these studies yielded prevalence rates for mental disorders that many observers consider much too high. This perception, rather than producing new pressure for greater mental health funding to respond to the discovered unmet need, has thrown into doubt the credibility of psychiatric epidemiology itself as a valid indicator of true prevalence and as a guide to policy formation. Second, the two aforementioned studies, despite very similar methods and levels of sophistication and rigor (albeit using somewhat different criteria from different editions of the DSM), yielded prevalence estimates that often are very far apart for the same disorder, again suggesting some problem with the validity of one or both sets of criteria. The evidence from psychiatric epidemiology thus seems to indicate that some changes need to be made in DSM definitions of disorders to achieve greater validity of the criteria.

It is propitious that this crisis in epidemiology comes at the time when psychiatry is starting to focus on a major revision to DSM-IV. (A text revision was published in 2000 [American Psychiatric Association 2000].) There is a common observation that the Chinese character for "crisis" is the same as the one for "opportunity." In this case, epidemiology's crisis is DSM's opportunity to learn something of use for the revision process. Regier and Narrow (Chapter 2 of this volume) suggest that we take this opportunity to use what we have learned in epidemiology to redefine DSM disorders to make the criteria yield more plausible prevalence rates when applied to community populations. Implicit in the Regier and Narrow chapter is the notion that changes in diagnostic criteria that would be useful for psychiatric epidemiology would also be useful for general clinical and research uses and should be part of the revision process leading to DSM-V. Thus, we approach the analysis of lessons from epidemiology with this broad goal in mind—that epidemiology will inform the process of developing DSM-V criteria that will be used in clinical and research settings, as well as in epidemiology.

The problem is in deciding exactly what we have learned from epidemiology. In Chapter 2, Regier and Narrow reanalyzed ECA and NCS data and demonstrated that, by adding a "clinical significance" criterion to the original DSM symptom criteria, lower and more reasonable prevalence rates are the result for a wide range of disorders. Furthermore, in the case of mood and anxiety disorders, Regier and Narrow argue that the addition of the clinical significance criterion leads to increased validity of diagnosis as evidenced by higher rates of service utilization and suicidal ideation or attempts. They suggest that this approach might be useful in revising DSM criteria.

It is easy in a variety of ways to add criteria to make diagnosis more demanding. The resulting lower prevalence estimates thus resolve the immediate problem of epidemiology's embarrassingly high levels of disorder. However, in the long run, what counts in redefining disorders—especially for clinical purposes—is not just lowering the prevalence rates to plausible levels but doing so in a way that is conceptually coherent and valid and serves the long-term interests of science and clinical practice. The fact that Regier and Narrow demonstrate that a clinical significance criterion added to diagnostic criteria lowers the prevalence rates does not demonstrate that this is the right way to achieve lower prevalence rates. The question is whether this method of lowering prevalence rates represents a valid redefinition of disorder that minimizes false positives as well as false negatives. In Chapter 2, Regier and Narrow offer no conceptual argument that their proposed solution is valid as an indicator of disorder and rely instead on the results of their data reanalysis.

In this chapter, we critically assess Regier and Narrow's proposal and the data analysis on which it is based. We proceed on the assumption that progress in diagnostic validity can be made only if there is a clear understanding of the relationships between disorder and the concepts of dysfunction, disability, and distress. We present a model of these relationships based on Wakefield's (1992, 1993) harmful dysfunction analysis of the concept of disorder. Once these relationships are clarified, it becomes evident that Regier and Narrow's proposals are problematic and that their data reanalyses of the ECA and NCS, although of interest in their own right, do not support the validity of their proposed strategy. Finally, we suggest an alternative approach to dealing with the seemingly excessively high community prevalence rates of mental disorders.

BASIC CONCEPTS

Although we cannot engage in a full analysis of the concept of *disorder* in this chapter, we offer a brief definition based on DSM-IV's definition of mental disorder (American Psychiatric Association 1994, pp. 21–22) as well as Wakefield's "harmful dysfunction" analysis. A basic assumption is that the concept of disorder as applied to psychiatric disorder is the same concept as that applied to general medical disorders. Simply put, all disorders (mental as well as physical) are conditions in which some function in the individual is not working as expected and, as a result, the individual is at risk of experiencing some form of harm—typically but not always in the form of distress or disability. Thus, for example, mood disorders represent a dysfunction of mood regulation, and, as a result, the individual experiences the distress of depressed mood or impairment in expected roles or usual activities. Note that *dysfunction* in the sense intended in this chapter refers to the failure of some internal mechanism in the person to perform a natural function (e.g., mood regulation in mood disorders, cognitive function in dementia, respiratory function in asthma).

In this chapter, *distress* refers to consciously perceived painful affects that are intrinsic to a condition; simply being distressed about having a condition is not included. Thus, people who are overweight or have unusually large noses may be distressed by these conditions, but the distress is not intrinsic to the condition. On the other hand, headaches and angina involve intrinsically distressing symptoms. Similarly anxiety, whether normal or pathological, is intrinsically distressing.

By *disability*, we mean the extent to which a condition interferes with socially expected roles or usual activities. Like distress, this interference varies on a continuum from some difficulty in carrying out usual activities to complete inability to carry out essential life activities.

Although most mental (and physical) disorders in extreme form are associated with distress and disability, the overall conceptual relationship is quite complex, as illustrated in Figure 3-1. The cells in the Venn diagram are illustrated by the following examples.

The A cell represents disorders with both distress and disability. Most severe mental (and physical) disorders fall under this category. Examples of these disorders include schizophrenia, in which psychotic symptoms typically impair social and occupational functioning and cause the patient extreme distress; depressive disorders that involve painful affect and that impair the ability to carry out everyday activities; and panic disorder with agoraphobia in which there is extreme distress (panic attacks) and impaired ability to carry on daily functioning.

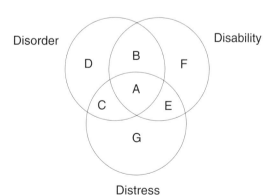

FIGURE 3-1   Relationship between disorder, distress, and disability. A = disorders with distress and disability; B = disorders with disability but no distress; C = disorders with distress but no disability; D = disorders with no distress and no disability; E = nondisorders with distress and disability; F = nondisorders with disability but no distress; G = nondisorders with distress but no disability.

The B cell represents disorders with disability but no distress. For example, antisocial personality disorder by definition involves impairment in social functioning (disability) yet often it is not accompanied by any distress. Similarly, a learning-disabled child will be impaired in academic functioning (disability) but will not necessarily experience distress.

The C cell represents disorders with distress but no disability. Many individuals with mood and anxiety disorders, even when the disorder is rather severe, have sufficient ego strength or stoicism such that the distressing symptoms do not keep them from carrying out usual activities.

The D cell represents disorders with no distress and no disability. Examples include some of the paraphilias. For example, many individuals with pedophilia experience no distress from the condition, nor do they find that it interferes with their ability to carry out usual activities (disability). An example from child psychiatry is some tic disorders in which the child is neither distressed by the tic nor affected by it in his or her usual activities.

The E cell represents nondisorders with distress and disability. The most commonly cited example is normal grief (DSM's uncomplicated bereavement), which is always associated with distress and frequently—at least temporarily—causes inability to function in normal social roles (disability). Other examples include transient but appropriate intense anxiety or depression in response to a major life event.

The F cell represents nondisorders with disability but no distress. Examples include illiteracy and some forms of subculturally sanctioned antisocial behavior (e.g., child and adolescent antisocial behavior associated with membership in a gang).

The G cell represents nondisorders with distress but no disability. Examples include unhappiness over negative life events and anxiety about real dangers.

Clinical significance criteria often require distress or impairment (disability) or both. Distress or disability or both is neither necessary nor sufficient for disorder. Failure to understand this fact prevents the formulation of a valid solution to the problem of false positives in psychiatric epidemiology.

PROBLEMS WITH REGIER AND NARROW'S CLINICAL SIGNIFICANCE CRITERION AS A VALIDATOR OF DISORDER STATUS

As Regier and Narrow's tables in Chapter 2 indicate, when the clinical significance criterion is added to the symptomatic criteria used in the epidemiologic studies, prevalence rates are reduced as expected. The issue that remains to be considered is how successful this approach is in excluding only false positives and not excluding any true positives. In psychiatric epidemiology, it is possible that prevalence rates might be made closer to true prevalence by changes in criteria that yield approximately equal rates of false positives and false negatives. However, in clinical settings, such tradeoffs should be avoided if at all possible.

As Regier and Narrow note, DSM-IV added a clinical significance criterion to many of the criteria sets in an effort to minimize false positives. Although Regier and Narrow use the same term, *clinical significance*, for the criterion that is added to the symptomatic criteria in their reanalyses, it should be noted that their clinical significance criteria are quite different from those in DSM-IV. In general, the DSM-IV clinical significance criterion requires that "the symptoms cause clinically significant distress or impairment in social, occupational, or other important areas of functioning." In contrast, Regier and Narrow's criteria include a disability question ("Did the symptoms interfere with your life or activities a lot?") and several questions concerning service utilization (e.g., "Did you tell a doctor about your symptoms?" "Did you take medicine for your symptoms more than once?" "Did you ever see a mental health specialist about your symptoms?"). Thus, whereas the DSM-IV clinical significance criterion requires either distress or disability, Regier and Narrow's clinical significance criterion requires either disability or service utilization and does not explicitly evaluate distress, although service utilization may be a partial indirect indicator of distress.

There are several problems with Regier and Narrow's strategy of using service utilization as a validator of disorder. First, it is ironic that Regier and Narrow seek to preserve the credibility of psychiatric epidemiology by using service utilization as a validator of disorder. The main motive for psychiatric epidemiologic studies of community populations is to measure the prevalence of disorder independently of service use by going beyond those who are identified as patients. A second problem is that many people with nondisorders seek services, making service use an ineffective validator of disorder for the purpose of eliminating false positives. Similarly, many people tell their doctors about various problems they are having that may not be due to disorders. As DSM-IV makes clear in its discussion of the V codes, nondisorders can appropriately require professional attention from a mental health professional. A third problem arises from Regier and Narrow's attempt to validate their clinical significance criterion by evaluating whether the addition of the criterion increases the rate of service utilization. Thus, a sample partly defined by service utilization is found to have higher service utilization—a tautology.

Regier and Narrow's use of disability as a validator of disorder also presents several problems. First, there is the problem of using disability to eliminate false positives. As Figure 3-1 shows, nondisorders may be associated with disability. In fact, Regier et al. (1998) correctly noted: "Based on the high prevalence rates identified in both the ECA and the NCS, it is reasonable to hypothesize that some syndromes in the community represent transient homeostatic responses to internal or external stimuli that do not represent true psychopathologic disorders" (p. 114). This corresponds to our E, F, or G cells in the figure. These deviations from homeostasis are precisely the kinds of normal conditions in which marked distress and social and role disabilities are likely to occur. Thus, Regier and Narrow's disability criterion is not effective in eliminating false positives of the kind that Regier suggested may be at the root of psychiatric epidemiology's problems.

Second, as we have noted, some psychiatric disorders, such as depression or anxiety disorders, may not be associated with any significant disability at all, so the disability criterion almost certainly will result in false negatives. In a classic article, "The Clinician's Illusion," Cohen and Cohen (1984) noted the tendency of clinicians to mistakenly assume that all individuals with a disorder are as disabled as the individuals they see in clinical practice. How often individuals in the community have true mental disorders yet are neither disabled nor seek professional help remains unknown and should be the object of epidemiologic study; instead, Regier and Narrow's approach in their reanalyses arbitrarily defines this population out of existence.

Third, Regier and Narrow require that the problem interfer with life or activities "a lot." Such a high threshold for disability eliminates people who only have mild or moderate disability from the disorder category. People with mild or moderate disability are not necessarily false positives; just as in general medicine, disorders can be mild or moderate in their effects on functioning and still be disorders. Reducing prevalence rates by redefining disorder to eliminate conditions with mild or moderate impact on social functioning is not a useful way to improve the validity of psychiatric epidemiology. Certainly this approach is not acceptable clinically because it gives rise to many false negatives.

On conceptual grounds, it can be argued that Regier and Narrow's clinical significance criterion is likely to eliminate some true cases of disorder and thus is likely to give rise to false negatives, in addition to failing to eliminate many false positives. An examination of their data suggests that this is almost certainly the case. Table 2-9, "Validity Indicators: Any Anxiety Disorder and Unipolar Major Depression," indicates that in both the ECA and NCS a significant number of individuals who met the symptomatic criteria for major depression but did not meet the clinical significance criterion nevertheless reported suicidal ideation or suicide attempts. Granting that not all suicidal ideation or attempts represent disorder, it is difficult to avoid the conclusion that some or perhaps even most of these cases are likely to involve individuals with depressive disorders for which they did not seek help and which they did not report to interfere with their lives "a lot."

ALTERNATIVE SUGGESTIONS FOR SOLVING THE FALSE-POSITIVE PROBLEM

We agree with Regier and Narrow that the false-positive problem in psychiatric diagnosis is a real one and that it should be addressed in the development of DSM-V. As we have argued elsewhere (Spitzer and Wakefield 1999; Wakefield 1996, 1997), the solution is to carefully examine and revise each criteria set rather than add a generic clinical significance criterion, however defined. Moreover, both the DSM-IV clinical significance criterion and Regier and Narrow's clinical significance criterion fail to address what we suspect is the major source of false positives in psychiatric epidemiologic studies—namely, the failure to exclude normal symptomatic conditions that occur in response to negative environmental circumstances. This view of false positives is consistent with Regier's own comment noted previously that false positives are often due to transient and normal deviations from homeostasis. To eliminate such normal deviations from homeostasis from the disorder category, the social context in which the symptoms occur must be taken into account because the very same clinically significant symptoms can be caused by an internal dysfunction or can be a normal response to extreme environmental stressors. Social context factors are not addressed in DSM-IV, nor are they addressed in Regier and Narrow's approaches to eliminating false positives by clinical significance criteria. Moreover, individuals with normal deviations from homeostasis may experience marked distress and impairment in social functioning, may consider the condition to interfere with their lives or activities "a lot," and may mention the problem to or seek help with the problem from a medical or mental health professional. Thus, such cases may end up being false positives even after the addition of Regier and Narrow's or DSM-IV's clinical significance criterion.

What is needed to deal with the false-positive problem is some kind of "social context" exclusion clause tailored to each diagnostic category where appropriate. The idea, in accordance with DSM-IV's definition of disorder and Wakefield's harmful dysfunction analysis of the concept of disorder, is to eliminate those conditions that are not a result of a dysfunction in the person. For example, in the case of major depression, such a criterion might be: "The symptoms are not simply a proportional and appropriate response to negative life circumstances or events." Of course, excluding normative responses to negative life circumstances does not deny that sometimes negative circumstances are so overwhelming that they do cause a dysfunction in the individual and thus cause a disorder. In such cases, the response is no longer proportional and appropriate to the life circumstances. This alternative approach to dealing with the false-positive problem, including reanalysis of ECA and NCS data by using this approach, is currently being undertaken by the senior author (J.C.W.) of this chapter.

COLLECTING DISABILITY DATA IN PSYCHIATRIC EPIDEMIOLOGY STUDIES

Although we have criticized the use of disability to eliminate false-positive diagnoses, we agree with Regier and Narrow about the practical importance of disability in considering policy implications of epidemiologic data. However, disability should be considered an independent dimension. There are two ways in which disability could be considered independently. First, for each mental disorder diagnosis, there could be an additional rating of the extent to which that disorder caused a certain degree of disability. The problem with this approach is that it becomes extremely difficult for a subject with several disorders (e.g., alcoholism, depression, a personality disorder) to disentangle the exact degree of impairment that separately can be attributed to each disorder. The second and more practical approach is to have an overall rating of disability due to mental disorder for the individual. This approach has the advantage that disability is not confused with disorder; yet policymakers and other consumers of epidemiologic data will have a useful indicator of service needs. For example, rather than just reporting the prevalence of anxiety disorders in the community, it would be possible to report the prevalence of both anxiety disorders in general and anxiety disorders in individuals with at least moderate disability. Moreover, normal but possibly disabling anxiety responses to real environmental threats and challenges, which may also be linked to service use, could now be reported in categories corresponding to the V codes in DSM.

CONCLUSIONS

Any approach to solving the false-positive problem in psychiatric epidemiology cannot ignore the conceptual issues involved in distinguishing disorders from nondisorders and must recognize that disorder, disability, and distress are complexly related concepts. Regier and Narrow's solution does not adequately address the false-positive problem in epidemiology and would cause potentially serious problems if applied to clinical practice. If the kinds of conceptual distinctions we noted are to be taken seriously, then there is an urgent need for research on possible false positives that meet current DSM symptomatic criteria. This area of research has been totally neglected, yet it is critical when considering revisions to DSM criteria. Conceptual and empirical research on this question should be undertaken to serve as a basis for proposals to revise the DSM criteria to improve their validity.

REFERENCES

American Psychiatric Association: Diagnostic and Statistical Manual of Mental Disorders, 4th Edition. Washington, DC, American Psychiatric Association, 1994

American Psychiatric Association: Diagnostic and Statistical Manual of Mental Disorders, 4th Edition, Text Revision. Washington, DC, American Psychiatric Association, 2000

Cohen P, Cohen J: The clinician's illusion. Arch Gen Psychiatry 41:1178–1182, 1984

Kessler RC, McGonagle KA, Zhao S, et al: Lifetime and 12-month prevalence of DSM-III-R psychiatric disorders in the United States: results from the National Comorbidity Survey. Arch Gen Psychiatry 51:8–19, 1994

Regier DA, Kaelber CT, Rae DS, et al: Limitations of diagnostic criteria and assessment instruments for mental disorders: implications for research and policy. Arch Gen Psychiatry 55:109–115, 1998

Robins LN, Regier DA (eds): Psychiatric Disorders in America. New York, Free Press, 1991

Spitzer RL, Wakefield JC: DSM-IV diagnostic criterion for clinical significance: does it help solve the false positives problem? Am J Psychiatry 156:1856–1864, 1999

Wakefield JC: The concept of mental disorder: on the boundary between biological facts and social values. Am Psychol 47:373–388, 1992

Wakefield JC: Disorder as harmful dysfunction: a conceptual critique of DSM-III-R's definition of mental disorder. Psychol Rev 99:232–247, 1993

Wakefield JC: DSM-IV: are we making diagnostic progress? Contemporary Psychology 41:646–652, 1996

Wakefield JC: Diagnosing DSM-IV—Part 1: DSM-IV and the concept of disorder. Behav Res Ther 35: 633–649, 1997

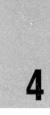

4

Psychometric Perspectives on Comorbidity

Robert F. Krueger, Ph.D.

Professionals who provide clinical services and undertake research intended to help persons with mental disorders were often taught that, in assessing our patients, we should strive to assign the most correct, single diagnosis. The concept typically invoked here is *differential diagnosis*, which involves carefully considering all possible diagnoses and picking the one that best accounts for the data gathered throughout the clinical interview. Consider, for example, how this approach is embodied in the text (Morrison 1995) I use in a course I teach on clinical interviewing. Morrison, the author of the text, provides students with a set of "rational diagnostic rules" as "a tool for thinking rationally about patients, even if their symptoms are confusing or contradictory" (p. 205). The second of these rules is "the fewer the diagnoses, the better." Although multiple diagnoses are sometimes warranted, this scenario is meant to be the exception, not the rule.

Despite this tradition of parsimony in the diagnosis of mental disorders, the idea that persons with one mental disorder often have others—the concept of *comorbidity*—has spread throughout the psychopathology literature (Lilienfeld et al. 1994). The comorbidity concept originated in literature on the epidemiology of medical diseases and was defined by Feinstein

(1970) as "any distinct additional entity that has existed or that may occur during the clinical course of a patient who has the index disease under study" (p. 467). Similarly, Blashfield (1990), writing about comorbidity in the psychopathological literature, noted that "comorbidity is a term from medicine that refers to the co-occurrence of different diseases in the same individual" (p. 61). Thus, comorbidity, as defined originally with reference to medical conditions and applied more recently to psychopathological conditions, refers to the idea that different diseases have co-occurred in the same person.

The constructs that psychopathologists use in their research and clinical work are often viewed as different diseases, in the sense intended by these definitions of comorbidity. In this way, comorbidity among mental disorders (such as those described in DSM) is meant to describe the situation in which distinct, additional diseases co-occur in the same person. How often do DSM-defined mental disorders co-occur? Is this scenario as rare as suggested by Morrison's "rational diagnostic rule"?

MAGNITUDE OF PSYCHOPATHOLOGICAL COMORBIDITY

Extensive evidence suggests that comorbidity is, in fact, far from rare. Indeed, in many situations, comorbidity appears to be more the rule than the exception (Clark et al. 1995). Although this finding is not new (Angst et al. 1990; Boyd et al. 1984; Sturt 1981), because of space limitations, I focus on evidence from the most recent large-scale survey of mental disorders in the United States—the National Comorbidity Survey (NCS; Kessler et al. 1994).

In the NCS, 79% of all lifetime mental disorders occurred in persons who met criteria for at least one other lifetime mental disorder. In other words, the majority of lifetime mental disorders are experienced by persons who have already revealed a propensity toward mental disorder. Moreover, this concentration of mental disorders in persons who have experienced other mental disorders is not limited to lifetime mental disorders. In the NCS, 59% of past-year disorders occurred in the 14% of the sample with a lifetime history of three or more mental disorders. Put differently, more than one-half of all past-year disorders were concentrated in the 14% of the sample that was already carrying a heavy burden of mental disorder. These data are a striking counterpoint to Morrison's "rational diagnostic rule." They suggest that comorbidity is far from rare and, moreover, that most recent (i.e., past-year) cases have rather complex, multifaceted histories of mental disorder.

CONCEPTUAL CONCERNS REGARDING THE COMORBIDITY CONCEPT AS APPLIED TO PSYCHOPATHOLOGICAL CONDITIONS

Perhaps Morrison's "rational diagnostic rule" is in need of revision, and we need to develop strategies for understanding and treating "multimorbid" persons. But is "comorbidity" the best concept for understanding the empirical data on patterns of co-occurrence among mental disorders? The extensive data on patterns of co-occurrence among mental disorders in population-based samples, as well as my experiences in working in clinical settings, led me to question the appropriateness of the comorbidity concept as typically applied to psychopathology. In clinical settings, I found myself evaluating and working with patients with "confusing and contradictory" presentations more often than seemed reasonable, given what I was led to expect about the frequency of "pure" cases. It seemed that the 14% of the U.S. population with lifetime histories of three or more mental disorders, as well as a current mental disorder, were precisely the persons whom I was being asked to evaluate, assign a "single most appropriate diagnosis" to, and treat. I have therefore been forced to grapple directly with the "comorbidity" phenomenon not only in pursuing research on mental disorders but also in attempting to conceptualize and help people with a complex mix of both current and historical problems. Considerations from research and from my clinical work have led me to the following broad concerns about the appropriateness of the comorbidity concept as typically applied to psychopathology. These concerns fall into three basic areas: person-level, variable-level, and research-design.

Person-Level Concerns

Definitions of comorbidity reveal it to be a person-level concept (Blashfield 1990; Feinstein 1970). Comorbidity refers to the co-occurrence of diseases within persons; that is, the concept suggests that two distinct diseases have co-occurred in the same person. The problem with this concept as applied to individuals with psychopathological conditions is that "trimorbid," "quadramorbid," and so on, persons are often encountered in clinical settings (Clark et al. 1995). Yet the way we think about treatment is still heavily influenced by the notion that a careful differential diagnosis will lead us to the correct label for which we should apply the corresponding treatment.

To a certain extent, the influence of a one-disorder, one-corresponding-treatment approach is waning as the reality of comorbidity is being increasingly recognized. We now see the emergence of programs for the treatment

of "dual-diagnosis" persons and the exploration of novel treatment strategies for patients with comorbidity (Wetzler and Sanderson 1997). Certainly,
given data suggesting that comorbidity is far from rare, these are welcome
developments. But these developments still may not capture the real meaning of the comorbidity phenomenon. Along these lines, evidence from treatment research suggests that many interventions are relatively nonspecific
and are useful in treating a variety of psychopathological conditions. Consider, for example, treatments for putatively separate unipolar affective and
anxiety disorders. Many conditions in this realm respond positively to selective serotonin reuptake inhibitors (SSRIs; Dunner 1998; Oehrberg et al.
1995; Ravindran et al. 1994). Moreover, this nonspecificity of response
is not limited to psychopharmacologic interventions. Psychosocial interventions in this realm also exhibit nonspecificity of response (Borkovec
et al. 1995; Brown et al. 1995). One possible implication of treatment nonspecificity is that treatments may be affecting core processes that underlie
and unite putatively separate mental disorders, spanning a range of both
normal and abnormal variation. Consider evidence that the SSRI paroxetine reduces levels of negative affectivity in normal research participants
(i.e., persons without a lifetime history of mental disorder themselves or in
their first-degree relatives; Knutson et al. 1998). If these findings prove to be
replicable, they suggest that unipolar affective and anxiety disorders may
be usefully reconceptualized as extreme variants on the temperamental
theme of negative affect. Comorbidity may be trying to show us that many
current treatments are not so much treatments for transient "state" mental
disorders of affect and anxiety as they are treatments for core processes,
such as negative affectivity, that span normal and abnormal variation as
well as undergird multiple mental disorders.

Variable-Level Concerns

Another concern about the comorbidity concept as applied to psychopathological conditions involves the mapping of the concept onto empirical
data regarding relations among diagnostic variables. It is not unusual to
encounter reports of comorbidity in the literature in which the authors report that "X% of all cases evaluated were comorbid, i.e., X% of cases met
criteria for disorders A and B." Such reports are not especially informative
because the percentage of all cases with both disorders (i.e., the percentage
of cases that were comorbid) provides only a portion of the information
useful in evaluating the data (Angold et al. 1999). A notable percentage of
cases with both disorders could be observed under different scenarios—
knowing the percentage of cases with both disorders does not allow us to

sort out these scenarios. For example, a notable percentage of comorbid cases could be the result of both disorders having high prevalence rates (or "base rates"). Consider a situation in which both disorders have a base rate of 50% (i.e., one-half the participants meet criteria for A and one-half the participants meet criteria for B). Simply by chance, we would expect to observe a notable percentage of participants with both conditions (25%) because the joint probability of two independent events (A and B) is equal to the probability of A (0.5) multiplied by the probability of B (0.5).

However, what if the disorders co-occur at greater-than-chance levels? This idea, that disorders might co-occur at greater-than-chance levels, is the concept of *correlation*; that is, if we observe more comorbid cases than we would expect by chance, the disorders should be said to be correlated. Put differently, two diagnostic variables are correlated if the two disorders co-occur at rates greater than the product of the base rates of the two disorders.

I do not think we can blame the authors for reports that give the percentage of cases with both disorders for confusing co-occurrence and correlation. The problem does not lie with these authors—who have faithfully applied the comorbidity concept to their data—but with the concept itself. The comorbidity concept fails to adequately distinguish between co-occurrence and correlation, even though these are distinct concepts with distinct implications. Comorbidity, as defined, means that people who meet criteria for more than one disorder may sometimes be observed (i.e., some people have two disorders that have co-occurred). From this standpoint, the percentage of cases where the disorders co-occurred answers the question, "how many cases were comorbid cases?" However, as we have seen, the observation that "X% of cases are comorbid" does not allow us to distinguish between co-occurrence and correlation. However, this distinction is crucial in making sense of the empirical data on "comorbidity." Consider, for example, the NCS data, which suggest a tendency for new mental disorders to occur disproportionately in persons with an already-manifested propensity toward mental disorders. The implication of this statement is that the diagnostic variables derived from DSM are signaling a phenomenon richer than can be captured by the comorbidity concept. The implication is, in fact, that the DSM variables are signaling patterns of correlation among mental disorders.

Research-Design Concerns

The tendency for disorders to be correlated also creates serious problems in implementing classical experimental psychopathology research designs (Clark et al. 1995). By classical research designs, I am referring to designs in which persons who meet criteria for a diagnosis are compared with persons (typically matched on demographic variables such as age and gender) who do not meet criteria for the diagnosis and, sometimes, also with persons who meet criteria for a different diagnosis. This type of design makes sense if mental disorders are relatively mutually exclusive. However, evidence of extensive correlations among DSM variables challenges the assumption of mutual exclusivity of disorders. Indeed, given significant correlations among multiple disorders, an investigator is faced with two rather problematic strategies for conducting research within the classical experimental psychopathology paradigm.

First, the investigator could try to recruit "pure" cases for his or her research—that is, persons who meet criteria for only the disorder of interest and not for other disorders. Given the extent of comorbidity among disorders, pursuing the pure-groups strategy is often frustrating and difficult. Moreover, pure cases are often rare relative to comorbid cases (Wittchen et al. 1999); hence, research with pure cases may not generalize to the population of all persons meeting criteria for the disorder of interest.

Second, the investigator could pursue an "impure" groups or "all-comers" strategy in which all persons who meet criteria for the target disorder are invited to participate, regardless of the comorbid disorders for which they might meet criteria. The patterns of comorbidity observed within the group of persons meeting criteria for the target disorder could be described in a table alongside the main findings from the study. Although this strategy should yield findings applicable to the population of persons meeting criteria for the disorder of interest, it suffers from its own problems. Specifically, because many persons with the target disorder have secondary disorders, it is difficult to determine whether the target disorder—rather than a secondary disorder or even a specific combination of target and secondary disorders (Sher and Trull 1996)—is driving the findings. Moreover, the pattern of secondary disorders may differ across studies, making replication across different research groups difficult.

PSYCHOMETRIC SOLUTION: COMORBIDITY SIGNALS MEANINGFUL PATTERNS OF CORRELATION

Given these person-level, variable-level, and research-design concerns, I have undertaken research in which I have tried to understand "comorbidity" as a signal of meaningful patterns of correlation among putatively separate mental disorders. The idea is that specific mental disorders described in DSM may be conceived of as *facets* (i.e., correlated subcomponents) of broad, underlying dimensions of psychopathological variation. The goal of this research is to try to detect the signatures of these broad, underlying dimensions by examining patterns of correlations among DSM-derived diagnostic variables.

In taking this approach, I have relied on tools and concepts from psychometrics and differential psychology. I turned to these fields because investigators in these areas have developed statistical techniques useful in modeling patterns of correlations among directly observed variables in terms of a smaller number of latent (not directly observed) variables. These tools and concepts are useful in the study of individual-difference variables such as personality and intelligence. Although they have also been used in studying psychopathology, research on psychopathology from a psychometric perspective has proceeded mostly independently of research on psychopathology from a more categorical or neo-Kraepelinian perspective (Blashfield 1984). Nevertheless, there is nothing inherent in psychometric techniques that prevents their use in studying neo-Kraepelinian constructs; by applying psychometric techniques to the comorbidity phenomenon, it is possible to fuse these two historically separate streams of research on the classification of psychopathology.

In particular, the psychometric technique of confirmatory factor analysis (CFA) has figured prominently in my work on modeling patterns of correlations among mental disorders. CFA is a formal statistical means of explaining associations among observed variables using a smaller number of unobserved, or latent, variables. In this work, CFA has been applied to tetrachoric correlations among DSM-defined mental disorder diagnoses derived from structured interviews. The *tetrachoric correlation* is the correlation between two dichotomous variables under the assumption that the observed dichotomies resulted from the setting of cutpoints on normally distributed latent continua. In psychiatric genetics, this model has been described as the *liability-threshold model* (Falconer 1965). The normally distributed variable underlying an observed, dichotomous diagnosis is the *liability* to experience the disorder. The cut point on the liability, above which persons meet criteria for the diagnosis, is the *threshold*. The appropriateness of the liability-threshold model and the tetrachoric correlation have been supported in research on numerous common mental disorders (Kendler 1993).

FINDINGS FROM A PSYCHOMETRIC PERSPECTIVE

I focus here on findings from two samples, the Dunedin Multidisciplinary Health and Development Study (DMHDS; Silva and Stanton 1996) and the NCS. The DMHDS is a longitudinal study of the health, development, and behavior of a complete cohort born between April 1, 1972, and March 31, 1973, in Dunedin, a city on New Zealand's South Island. When the cohort members were 18 ($N = 930$) and 21 years old ($N = 937$), they were interviewed using the Diagnostic Interview Schedule (DIS, Version III-R; Robins et al. 1989) to obtain diagnoses of mental disorder in the previous 12 months. Diagnoses of major depressive episode, dysthymia, generalized anxiety disorder, agoraphobia, social phobia, simple phobia, obsessive-compulsive disorder, marijuana dependence, alcohol dependence, and conduct disorder were sufficiently prevalent for submission to CFA. At age 21, conduct disorder was replaced by the more age-appropriate diagnosis of antisocial personality disorder.

Various models for the structure of the 10 diagnoses were evaluated: a one-factor model in which all 10 diagnoses were presumed to reflect a single general psychopathology factor; a two-factor model in which the disorders were grouped into two broad classes—internalizing and externalizing; and a four-factor model in which the disorders were grouped into four broad classes—affective disorder, anxiety disorder, substance dependence, and antisocial behavior (Krueger et al. 1998). At both age 18 and age 21, the best-fitting model for these data was the two-factor, internalizing/externalizing model in which major depressive episode, dysthymia, generalized anxiety disorder, agoraphobia, social phobia, simple phobia, and obsessive-compulsive disorder were indicators of internalizing, and marijuana dependence, alcohol dependence, and conduct disorder/antisocial personality disorder were indicators of externalizing. The labels for these factors (internalizing/externalizing) were derived from work on empirically based psychopathological syndromes in childhood and adolescence (see Chapter 10, "Empirically Based Assessment and Taxonomy Across the Life Span," this volume). The empirically based approach works from the "bottom-up," using exploratory multivariate statistical techniques to determine how symptoms cohere to form syndromes, whereas the DSM approach works more from the "top-down," relying on expert consensus to determine the symptoms associated with specific disorders (Achenbach and McConaughy 1997). Yet both approaches converge on very similar broadband internalizing and externalizing factors. In addition, in our CFA models, the latent internalizing and externalizing factors were moderately intercorrelated (0.45 at age 18, 0.42 at age 21), as they are in data collected using Achenbach's instruments from his empirically based approach.

The design of the Dunedin study also allowed us to link the latent internalizing and externalizing factors across the two waves from age 18 to age 21. In modeling the data in this manner, we found substantial cross-time correlations: internalizing at age 18 was correlated 0.69 with internalizing at age 21, and externalizing at age 18 was correlated 0.86 with externalizing at age 21. These findings suggest that latent propensities toward mental disorder exhibit impressive differential (i.e., rank-order; Caspi and Bem 1990) stability over time. This finding is important because it suggests that a categorical perspective on the longitudinal stability of mental disorder diagnoses may sometimes be misleading. Although few persons may meet criteria for exactly the same diagnosis (or pattern of diagnoses) at two waves of a longitudinal study (Ollendick and King 1994), this apparent instability at the diagnostic category level disguises stability at the latent, broadband factor level.

The next task was to determine if these findings were replicable in other samples; thus I pursued analyses similar to those conducted in the Dunedin data in the NCS data (Krueger 1999b). As noted earlier, the NCS is the most recent large-scale survey of mental disorders in the United States, and these data allowed the model developed in the Dunedin data to be extended in key ways. The 8,098 NCS participants constituted a national probability sample of noninstitutionalized U.S. civilians ages 15 to 54 who were interviewed by trained nonclinician interviewers using the University of Michigan Composite International Diagnostic Interview (Kessler et al. 1994), which allowed participants to be given DSM-III-R diagnoses. Using the same statistical approach used for the Dunedin data, the best-fitting model for the NCS data was found to be a model in which major depressive episode, dysthymia, and generalized anxiety disorder loaded on a factor labeled "anxious-misery," and social phobia, simple phobia, agoraphobia, and panic disorder loaded on a factor labeled "fear." Anxious-misery and fear, in turn, loaded on a broad latent internalizing factor, which was again moderately correlated (0.51) with a latent externalizing factor, indicated by alcohol dependence, drug dependence, and antisocial personality disorder. The finding that this model fit the data best was replicated in random halves of the sample, in lifetime and past-year diagnoses, as well as separately in women and men. In a treatment-seeking subsample of the NCS, the best-fitting model collapsed anxious-misery and fear into one factor—internalization (i.e., the latent subfactors of internalization could not be distinguished in the treatment-seeking subsample).

INTERNALIZING AND EXTERNALIZING

At this point, it appears that internalizing and externalizing are replicable phenotypic dimensions undergirding patterns of correlations among common mental disorders. The basic pattern of findings has now been replicated across nations, genders, instruments, ages, and lifetime and past-year diagnoses. But what are the "inner natures" of the latent internalizing and externalizing variables? Is there evidence that these labels are psychologically meaningful? Research that my colleagues and I have undertaken on the personality correlates and predictors of mental disorders may be useful in fleshing out the psychological underpinnings of internalization and externalization. In our research, we relied on the model of personality traits developed by Tellegen (1985) and his instrument for measuring personality, the Multidimensional Personality Questionnaire (MPQ; Tellegen, in press). The MPQ measures a number of distinct personality traits that cohere in three broad, higher-order personality dimensions: positive emotionality (a low general threshold for the experience of positive emotions and enthusiastic engagement with the environment), negative emotionality (a low general threshold for the experience of negative emotions such as anxiety and anger), and constraint (a tendency to endorse social norms, act in a cautious and restrained manner, and avoid thrills). Members of the Dunedin birth cohort completed a version of the MPQ at age 18, and my colleagues and I reported on relationships between the MPQ and the DIS at ages 18 and 21 (Krueger et al. 1996). Briefly summarized, the Dunedin data suggest that negative emotionality is at the core of the four broad classes of common mental disorder. Persons from the Dunedin cohort who met criteria for affective, anxiety, substance dependence, and antisocial disorders were distinguished from persons free from disorder by high negative emotionality. Yet negative emotionality is not the only trait relevant to common mental disorders, because persons who met criteria for substance dependence and antisocial disorders could also be distinguished from persons free from disorder by their low levels of constraint.

I followed up these initial analyses with additional analyses in which the MPQ was used to predict changes in diagnostic status from age 18 to age 21 (Krueger 1999a). In these analyses, affective, anxiety, substance dependence, and antisocial behavior variables at age 21 were predicted by the MPQ at age 18, controlling for corresponding mental disorder variables at age 18. As noted earlier, there was substantial stability in mental disorder status from age 18 to age 21 (Krueger et al. 1998). Hence, these analyses represent a particularly stringent test of the idea that personality is causally linked to mental disorder, because they require personality to predict *changes* in mental disorder (i.e., variance in age 21 mental disorder that could not be predicted simply by knowing mental disorder status at age 18). Affective and anxiety disorders at age 21 were predicted by high negative emotionality, and substance dependence and antisocial disorders at age 21 were predicted by both high negative emotionality and low constraint. Thus, negative emotionality and constraint appear to be causally linked to mental disorder, as well as to the form mental disorder takes during the transition from late adolescence to early adulthood.

The MPQ results from Dunedin suggest that internalizing and externalizing are apt descriptors of the latent factors that undergird common DSM disorders. Both internalizing and externalizing disorders contain an element of distress (i.e., negative emotionality). If this propensity toward distress is paired with low constraint, the distress is expressed outwardly, externalized in the form of socially undesirable behaviors such as crime and dependence on illicit substances. However, without the contribution of low constraint, high levels of distress are expressed inwardly, internalized as unipolar affective and anxiety disorder.

CONCLUSION

The evidence described in this chapter suggests that comorbidity among common mental disorders can be understood as meaningful patterns of correlation. Rather than considering unipolar affective, anxiety, substance dependence, and antisocial behavior disorders as discrete and separate entities that may sometimes co-occur, the perspective outlined here views these constructs as correlated facets of broad, underlying dimensions of psychopathological variation. In this way, the naturally occurring patterns of correlation among the disorders are accommodated and modeled, rather than having to be controlled for or ignored.

The perspective on comorbidity developed in this chapter does *not* imply that the distinctions between various syndromes are unimportant. A psychometric perspective conceives of individual syndromes, such as those described in DSM, as facets (subcomponents) of broad dimensions. The broad-factor level of analysis and the facet level of analysis are complementary, rather than competing. Thus, a psychometric perspective is ecumenical; that is, it provides a way of bringing together "lumpers," who focus on connections among various mental disorders, and "splitters," who focus on distinctions among various mental disorders. Determining which level of analysis is appropriate for a particular situation is an empirical matter, and adopting a psychometric perspective on comorbidity can further empirical research into this matter. For example, rather than relying on the empirically problematic pure-group and all-comers strategies, clinical trials could be conducted on representative samples drawn from specific outpatient populations. If these samples are described and characterized in terms of their profile across various common psychopathological syndromes, as well as their levels on the broad internalizing and externalizing dimensions, the impact of an intervention could be assessed at both the specific-facet and the broad-factor levels. It is possible that some interventions (e.g., the SSRIs) exert their impact at the broad-factor level, whereas others may affect specific psychopathological facets. By conceiving of common psychopathologies in a psychometric fashion, these sorts of possibilities can be subjected to empirical scrutiny. Indeed, this conception suggests a novel perspective on persons with multiple, complex patterns of comorbid diagnoses. Rather than being confusing, such cases may be clarifying, as they represent the high poles of the internalizing and externalizing dimensions.

In summary, a psychometric perspective appears useful in making sense of comorbidity among common mental disorders. The internalization and externalization dimensions uncovered by psychometric analyses of DSM variables are psychologically compelling and hold promise as targets for continuing research. Hopefully, these dimensions will continue to demonstrate their utility in pointing us toward core processes underlying mental disorders as we work toward better defining psychopathology in the twenty-first century.

REFERENCES

Achenbach TM, McConaughy SH: Empirically Based Assessment of Child and Adolescent Psychopathology, 2nd Edition. Thousand Oaks, CA, Sage, 1997

Angold A, Costello EJ, Erkanli A: Comorbidity. J Child Psychol Psychiatry 40:57–87, 1999

Angst J, Vollrath M, Merikangas KR, et al: Comorbidity of anxiety and depression in the Zurich cohort study of young adults, in Comorbidity of Affective and Anxiety Disorders. Edited by Maser JD, Cloninger CR. Washington, DC, American Psychiatric Press, 1990, pp 123–137

Blashfield RK: The Classification of Psychopathology: Neo-Kraepelinian and Quantitative Approaches. New York, Plenum, 1984

Blashfield RK: Comorbidity and classification, in Comorbidity of Affective and Anxiety Disorders. Edited by Maser JD, Cloninger CR. Washington, DC, American Psychiatric Press, 1990, pp 61–82

Borkovec TD, Abel JL, Newman H: Effects of psychotherapy on comorbid conditions in generalized anxiety disorder. J Consult Clin Psychol 63:479–483, 1995

Boyd JH, Burke JD Jr, Gruenberg E, et al: Exclusion criteria of DSM-III: a study of co-occurrence of hierarchy-free syndromes. Arch Gen Psychiatry 41:983–989, 1984

Brown TA, Antony MM, Barlow DH: Diagnostic comorbidity in panic disorder: effect on treatment outcome and course of comorbid diagnoses following treatment. J Consult Clin Psychol 63:408–418, 1995

Caspi A, Bem DJ: Personality continuity and change across the life course, in Handbook of Personality: Theory and Research. Edited by Pervin LA. New York, Guilford, 1990, pp 549–575

Clark LA, Watson D, Reynolds S: Diagnosis and classification of psychopathology: challenges to the current system and future directions. Annu Rev Psychol 46:121–153, 1995

Dunner DL: The issue of comorbidity in the treatment of panic. Int Clin Psychophar-macol 13:S19–S24, 1998

Falconer DS: The inheritance of liability to certain diseases, estimated from the inci-dence among relatives. Ann Hum Genet 29:51–76, 1965

Feinstein AR: The pre-therapeutic classification of co-morbidity in chronic disease. J Chronic Dis 23:455–468, 1970

Kendler KS: Twin studies of psychiatric illness: current status and future directions. Arch Gen Psychiatry 50:905–915, 1993

Kessler RC, McGonagle KA, Zhao S, et al: Lifetime and 12-month prevalence of DSM-III-R psychiatric disorders in the United States: results from the National Comor-bidity Survey. Arch Gen Psychiatry 51:8–19, 1994

Knutson B, Wolkowitz OM, Cole SW, et al: Selective alteration of personality and social behavior by serotonergic intervention. Am J Psychiatry 155:373–379, 1998

Krueger RF: Personality traits in late adolescence predict mental disorders in early adulthood: a prospective-epidemiological study. J Pers 67:39–65, 1999a

Krueger RF: The structure of common mental disorders. Arch Gen Psychiatry 56:921–926, 1999b

Krueger RF, Caspi A, Moffitt TE, et al: Personality traits are differentially linked to mental disorders: a multitrait-multidiagnosis study of an adolescent birth cohort. J Abnorm Psychol 105:299–312, 1996

Krueger RF, Caspi A, Moffitt TE, et al: The structure and stability of common mental disorders (DSM-III-R): a longitudinal-epidemiological study. J Abnorm Psychol 107:216–227, 1998

Lilienfeld SO, Waldman ID, Israel AC: A critical examination of the use of the term and concept of comorbidity in psychopathology research. Clinical Psychology: Science and Practice 1:71–83, 1994

Morrison J: The First Interview: Revised for DSM-IV. New York, Guilford, 1995

Oehrberg S, Christiansen PE, Behnke K, et al: Paroxetine in the treatment of panic disorder: a randomised, double-blind, placebo-controlled study. Br J Psychiatry 167:374–379, 1995

Ollendick TH, King NJ: Diagnosis, assessment, and treatment of internalizing problems in children: the role of longitudinal data. J Consult Clin Psychol 62:918–927, 1994

Ravindran AV, Bialik RJ, Lapierre YD: Therapeutic efficacy of specific serotonin reup-take inhibitors (SSRIs) in dysthymia. Can J Psychiatry 39:21–26, 1994

Robins LN, Helzer JE, Cottler L, et al: Diagnostic Interview Schedule, Version III-R. Unpublished manuscript, St. Louis, MO, Washington University, 1989

Sher KJ, Trull TJ: Methodological issues in psychopathology research. Annu Rev Psy-chol 47:371–400, 1996

Silva PA, Stanton WR (eds): From Child to Adult: The Dunedin Multidisciplinary Health and Development Study. Auckland, New Zealand, Oxford University Press, 1996

Sturt E: Hierarchical patterns in the distribution of psychiatric symptoms. Psychol Med 11:783–794, 1981

Tellegen A: Structures of affect and personality and their relevance to assessing anxiety, with an emphasis on self-report, in Anxiety and the Anxiety Disorders. Edited by Tuma AH, Maser JD. Hillsdale, NJ, Erlbaum, 1985, pp 681–706

Tellegen A: Manual for the Multidimensional Personality Questionnaire. Minneapolis, MN, University of Minnesota Press (in press)

Wetzler S, Sanderson WC (eds): Treatment Strategies for Patients With Psychiatric Comorbidity. New York, Wiley, 1997

Wittchen HU, Lieb R, Wunderlich U, et al: Comorbidity in primary care: presentation and consequences. J Clin Psychiatry 60:29–36, 1999

PART II   IMAGING PSYCHOPATHOLOGY

5

Toward a Neuroanatomical Understanding of Psychiatric Illness

The Role of Functional Imaging

Jane Epstein, M.D.
Nancy Isenberg, M.D., M.P.H.
Emily Stern, M.D.
David Silbersweig, M.D.

The advent of functional neuroimaging technologies is perhaps the most important of several recent developments that promise to erode, if not eradicate, the classification of mind/brain disorders as either psychiatric or neurologic. This classification, although entrenched in contemporary American medicine, was absent at neurology's inception as a subspecialty in the nineteenth century, when physicians investigating mental and behavioral aspects of brain function (e.g., Pick, Kraeplin, Alzheimer) referred to themselves as neuropsychiatrists. In the following decades, a number of factors gave rise to a split between physicians treating disorders of mind and of brain. These included both controversy surrounding the theoretical possibility of localizing mental functions to specific neural substrates (Finger 1994), and the practical difficulty of doing so. Indeed, Freud's decision to confine his investigations to the mental arena occurred only after he abandoned an attempt to translate clinical observations of mental processes into neurologic terms, convinced that contemporary knowledge of neurophysiology did not allow for its accomplishment (Kandel 1998).

Following Freud, American psychiatrists continued to focus mainly on mental phenomena until the latter half of the twentieth century, when several pharmacologic agents were discovered to be effective in the treatment of psychosis, mania, depression, and anxiety. The subsequent ascendance of biological psychiatry renewed the field's focus on the brain as the seat of the mind. It engendered a systematic approach to the description of clinical syndromes, based on the disease model, which allowed for their empiric investigation and a focus on associated neurochemical abnormalities with clear relevance for pharmacologic treatment. Paradoxically, these very strengths of early biological psychiatry, combined with a lack of access to, or awareness of, research and methodologic developments occurring in allied fields, initially impeded the further characterization of the neural correlates of mental disorders.

Emerging data from the cognitive neurosciences reveal that specific cognitive, emotional, perceptual, and behavioral functions are mediated by specific brain regions or circuits that, when disrupted, give rise to clinical abnormalities in those functions. Conversely, biological abnormalities described at the level of neural systems, as opposed to that of neurochemistry, can be more readily associated with cognitive, emotional, perceptual, or behavioral disturbances described at the level of mind (see Epstein et al. 2001). These considerations suggest that a useful approach to investigating the biological correlates of mental dysfunction might focus on individual psychiatric symptoms, rather than on entire syndromes (as the former can be more readily described in terms of dysfunction of specific cognitive, emotional, perceptual, or behavioral functions), and on neural regions or circuits, rather than on neurochemicals. Thus, in the context of basic and clinical behavioral neuroscientific findings from related fields, functional neuroimaging techniques, which allow for in vivo measurement of localized, systems-level brain function associated with specific symptoms or disease states, hold great promise for the reintegration of psychiatry and neurology, mind and brain.

In the following sections, we provide a brief overview of current functional neuroimaging methods, give examples of their use to define systems-level pathophysiology associated with psychiatric symptoms, and discuss the implications of such work for the taxonomy, diagnosis, and treatment of mental disorders.

FUNCTIONAL NEUROIMAGING METHODS

Technologies

This brief overview of functional neuroimaging methods focuses on positron emission tomography (PET) and functional magnetic resonance imaging (fMRI) because of their localizing ability and prominence in recent neuropsychiatric research. Focal increases in neuronal activity associated with particular mental processes are accompanied by increases in neuronal metabolism, closely coupled increases in blood flow and volume, and specific changes in blood oxygenation within the same region. Functional imaging technologies measure these alterations to localize changes in neuronal activity associated with specific mental phenomena.

With PET, a small amount of a compound labeled with a positron-emitting radioisotope is injected into the subject and distributed in the body according to the biochemical characteristics of the tracer. The emitted positrons combine with electrons, resulting in their annihilation and the production of photons. These are registered by detectors in the PET scanner, allowing for the reconstruction of an image containing information about the amount of radioactivity emitted from each point in the brain. Fluorine-18–labeled 2-deoxy-D-glucose (^{18}F-FDG) is often used to provide a measure of glucose metabolism associated with neuronal activity (Raichle 1987). Because it produces an image integrated over approximately 30 minutes, it is not able to capture discrete mental events but can provide a robust measure of basal brain activity. Due to its briefer half-life, oxygen-15–labeled water ($H_2{}^{15}O$) is frequently used to provide multiple, repeated 10- to 30-second integrated measures of brain activity in contrasting mental/symptom states. Neurochemistry can also be examined using specific radioactively labeled ligands to measure, for example, receptor density, neurochemical or metabolic precursors, intermediates or products, and neurochemical effects of pharmacologic agents.

Magnetic resonance imaging (MRI) uses a magnetic field to align protons in body tissues and a pulse of radiofrequency (RF) waves to excite those protons, resulting in emission of an RF signal registered by a receiver coil. Gradients are applied to the magnetic field to obtain spatial information, and a Fourier transformation is used to convert the acquired data into a spatial image. The most widely used functional MRI method, blood oxygen level–dependent (BOLD) imaging (Kwong et al. 1992; Ogawa et al. 1992, 1993), images endogenous changes in blood oxygenation, rendering intravenous infusion of an exogenous substance unnecessary. When neuronal activity increases, both local blood flow and oxygen consumption increase. Because the increase in blood flow exceeds that in oxygen consumption (Fox and Raichle 1986), there is a net increase in oxygenated blood and a net decrease in deoxyhemoglobin, which is paramagnetic. This decrease results in a focal increase in signal intensity on the functional images.

A more recently developed set of fMRI techniques, arterial spin labeling (ASL), is based on a more direct measure of cerebral blood flow (CBF) and is therefore more amenable to quantitation (Fox and Raichle 1986; Wong et al. 1999; Yang et al. 1998). With ASL, two sets of images are obtained: one in which protons in the arterial blood that are flowing into the image slices of interest are magnetically labeled, and one in which they are not. Measurement of CBF is derived by comparing labeled versus unlabeled images in contrasting mental states. This arterial weighting (vs. venous-weighted BOLD deoxyhemoglobin changes) may provide slightly improved spatial localization, but the complexity of the process imposes some design constraints that have limited its use to date. Although fMRI has several advantages over PET, such as improved spatial and temporal resolution, absence of ionizing radiation, and wide availability, it is also limited by a spatially constrained and noisy scanning environment and by signal artifact at the base of the brain, where structures of neuropsychiatric interest lie.

Study Design

Most functional imaging studies have employed a block design, in which the subject is instructed to continuously and repeatedly perform a specific mental operation for 20–60 seconds at a time. Scans from epochs representing one cognitive steady-state condition are then contrasted with scans from a control condition. More recently, many investigators have used event-related designs, which allow for the detection of neural activity associated with multiple brief mental events. An event-related PET technique (Silbersweig et al. 1994) has overcome limitations in the temporal discrimination of PET by considering the dynamic, instantaneous nature of radiotracer input making up the PET measure (which is integrated over time). Event-related fMRI techniques (Rosen et al. 1998) take advantage of MRI's direct temporal resolution, considering the vascular response profile produced by each individual event.

There are several approaches to designating and probing the mental phenomenon of interest (Stern and Silbersweig 2001). Symptoms or mental states can be imaged directly as they occur—either spontaneously, as a result of controlled provocation or induction, or in response to relevant stimuli. Alternatively, specific tasks can be used to probe either neuropsychological functions or brain regions/circuits, which are hypothesized to be abnormal in a particular disorder. Because most tasks involve multiple cognitive, emotional, perceptual, or motor functions, an activation task will often result in neural activity in circuits other than those associated with the specific mental phenomenon of interest. To control for this activity, a second task may be designed that shares all functions except for the one of particular interest. When activation associated with the control task is subtracted from that associated with the activation task, the remaining activation pattern is believed to represent the function of interest (Posner et al. 1988). In addition to activation and control tasks, it can be helpful to include a "resting state" either as a further control condition or as an independent baseline state. An alternative experimental approach uses a parametric design. In this case, a variable of interest [e.g., memory load (Grasby et al. 1994) or symptom rating score (Liddle et al. 1992)] varies continuously within or across subjects, and a regression analysis is used to identify brain regions in which activity correlates with the changing values.

Image Processing and Analysis

Following data acquisition, multiple processing steps are required prior to statistical analysis. Once images are reconstructed, they are generally corrected for sources of noise in the signal, realigned to correct for head movement, and smoothed to enhance the signal-to-noise ratio. For each individual subject, functional images can be coregistered to that subject's structural MRI for anatomical reference. Images to be compared across subjects may undergo stereotactic normalization, in which they are transformed to a stereotactic coordinate space based on a common template (Mazziotta et al. 1995). Statistical analyses may be hypotheses led or data led. They may focus on brain regions of interest or consider all brain regions on the basis of individual volume elements, or voxels, corrected for multiple comparisons. Univariate statistics are often used to compare activity in a given brain region with itself across conditions or diagnoses. Multiple linear regression analysis may be performed, as exemplified by statistical parametric mapping (SPM) (Friston et al. 1995; Mazziotta et al. 1995; Worsley and Friston 1995), to identify condition or diagnosis effects, or their interactions, within the context of the General Linear Model. Multivariate analysis may also be applied to identify correlations or interactions among numerous brain regions across time and conditions (Buchel et al. 1999; McIntosh and Gonzalez-Lima 1994).

USE OF FUNCTIONAL NEUROIMAGING TO DEFINE SYSTEMS-LEVEL PATHOPHYSIOLOGY ASSOCIATED WITH PSYCHIATRIC SYMPTOMS

When attempting to identify the brain circuits underlying neuropsychiatric disorders, a symptom-oriented strategy can be particularly effective for a variety of reasons. As mentioned above, individual symptom states are more likely to map onto particular neural substrates than are heterogeneous descriptive syndromes. In addition, psychiatric symptoms, such as delusions, do not necessarily segregate with diagnostic categories, and may occur in different syndromes such as schizophrenia or affective disorders. Similarly, psychopharmacologic agents, such as neuroleptics, successfully treat particular symptoms, such as delusions, regardless of their setting (Arana and Hyman 1991). For these reasons, symptom-oriented studies may be more likely to provide direct, non-model-dependent, pathophysiologically meaningful data than studies that target a neuropsychological deficit hypothesized to underlie a particular syndrome. This latter approach, although not the focus of this chapter, is nevertheless widely used, effective, and complementary to the symptom-oriented strategy described here. Following are some examples, taken from our work and that of Rauch and colleagues, of this symptom-oriented strategy. These are intended to illustrate its potential, rather than to provide a full review of the relevant literature.

We employed the symptom-oriented approach to study hallucinations and delusions in schizophrenia, and tics in Tourette's syndrome, using $H_2^{15}O$ PET. The hallucinations and tics were "captured" in the course of spontaneous occurrence using the event-related PET technique, described above, which we developed and validated with colleagues from London for this purpose. Psychological and neurobiological functions that may be involved in the formation of paranoid delusions were probed using an activation task based on the emotional Stroop (see below), with contrasting symptom-specific words. Rauch and colleagues employed symptom provocation techniques to study brain regions associated with symptoms in obsessive-compulsive disorder (OCD), simple phobia (SP), and post-traumatic stress disorder (PTSD) using $C^{15}O_2$ PET. These examples of symptom-oriented work in schizophrenia, TS, and anxiety disorders complement the important affective disorder studies described by Drevets and colleagues in Chapter 6 of this volume. Accordingly, descriptions of our work on manic versus euthymic state changes in frontal-subcortical circuit activity can be found elsewhere (Blumberg et al. 1999; Blumberg et al. 2000).

Hallucinations

Our study of hallucinations (Silbersweig et al. 1995) was performed on six right-handed subjects with DSM-IV (American Psychiatric Association 1994) diagnoses of schizophrenia, paranoid type. Five of these subjects were experiencing frequent, classic auditory–verbal hallucinations despite receiving neuroleptic medication; the other subject, who was analyzed separately, was neuroleptic-naive and was experiencing frequent hallucinations in both visual and auditory modalities. For each of 22–25 scans performed in two study sessions, the subjects were instructed to press a button with their right thumb when they heard voices (which were usually accompanied by visions in the drug-naive subject). The timing and duration of each hallucination in relation to radiotracer delivery to the brain was logged by computer and used to derive a weighted score for each scan reflecting the contribution, to the image, of radiotracer deposition during hallucinations. An event-related count-rate correlational analysis (Silbersweig et al. 1994) was then performed on the images within the framework of pixel-by-pixel SPM (Friston et al. 1995) to locate the brain regions in which activity was highly correlated with the occurrence of hallucinations.

In the individual subject with visual and auditory–verbal hallucinations, the pattern of significantly increased brain activity included areas in bilateral (left > right) visual, auditory, and multimodal association cortices, areas specialized for higher-order visual perception, speech perception, and intermodal processing. The more extensive left-sided activations may reflect the dominance of that hemisphere for language. Neocortical activations were absent from the group analysis of the five subjects with auditory–verbal hallucinations but present (including temporoparietal auditory–linguistic association cortex) in each individual subject. This was probably due to intersubject variability in the precise location of these neocortical activations, perhaps reflecting individual differences in the content of hallucinations.

The pattern of significant shared activity in the group included bilateral thalami, bilateral hippocampi/parahippocampal gyri, right anterior cingulate, right ventral striatum, and left orbitofrontal cortex. Areas of activation extended into bilateral amygdalae and the right orbitofrontal cortex. The individual subject also displayed increased activity in left posterior cingulate, right parahippocampal gyrus, and right temporal pole, as well as decreased activity in orbitofrontal cortex. The thalamic activity is intriguing in light of the integrative and modulatory roles of thalamocortical circuits in the generation of perceptual experience (Llinas and Pare 1991; Manford and Andermann 1998). The extensive activity of limbic/paralimbic structures may reflect the emotional/motivational attributes of the hallucinatory experiences.

Tics

We used similar methodology to identify brain circuits associated with tics in Tourette's syndrome (Stern et al. 2000). With our same British colleagues, we studied six right-handed subjects with Tourette's syndrome and frequent motor and vocal tics. Tics were monitored with video cameras, as well as with a throat microphone and tape recorder. Information about the exact timing of the tics relative to radiotracer delivery to the brain was used to identify brain regions in which activity was highly correlated with tic occurrence.

The pattern of correlated increases in brain activity included primary motor and language cortices (including Broca's area) corresponding to the modality-specific outflow pathways of behavioral expression in motor and vocal tics. Subcortically, increases were noted in striatal regions, consistent with the emphasis on basal ganglia circuits in traditional pathophysiologic models of Tourette's syndrome, and in midbrain tegmentum, a region containing the cell bodies of dopaminergic neurons involved in the modulation of such striato-pallido-thalamo-cortical circuits. Extensive increases were also detected in executive motor cortices (supplementary motor, premotor, anterior cingulate, and dorsolateral prefrontal)—areas involved in the selection, preparation, and initiation of behavior—perhaps reflecting the disordered action and volition associated with Tourette's syndrome.

Delusions

In contrast to the more "bottom-up" symptom capture paradigm used in the investigation of hallucinations and tics, we employed a "top-down" paradigm to probe psychological and neurobiological functions that may be involved in the formation of paranoid delusions (Epstein et al. 1999). Subjects were six DSM-IV schizophrenic subjects with active paranoid delusions, five DSM-IV schizophrenic subjects without active paranoid delusions, and six normal control subjects.

A variant of the emotional Stroop task, in which subjects were instructed to name the colors of neutral and interpersonal threat words, was used to test the hypothesis that mesolimbic activity in paranoid subjects who were processing neutral stimuli would resemble that seen in control subjects who were processing threatening stimuli. The task had previously been shown to differentiate behaviorally between actively and nonactively paranoid subjects with schizophrenia, with the former showing significantly increased reaction times to interpersonal threat words. Subjects were scanned within a block design while naming the colors of neutral words and interpersonal threat words and while resting. Images were analyzed using SPM, with evaluation of predefined contrasts for hypothesis testing.

In control subjects, interpersonal threat words were associated with amygdalar activation. A similar pattern of increased mesotemporal (periamygdalar/anterior parahippocampal) activity was observed in paranoid subjects compared with control subjects, even with neutral words. A double dissociation in right parahippocampal and ventral striatal activity was seen with semanto-linguistic threat, with increases noted in paranoid subjects, and decreases in control subjects. In paranoid subjects, a decrease in dorsal anterior cingulate activity was detected, with failure to modulate with task performance, whereas ventral frontal activity decreased on task in comparison with control subjects. This pattern of findings, somewhat akin to that seen in the study of hallucinations, suggests an increased, abnormally contextualized assignment of emotional relevance by amygdalar and hippocampal structures, unmodulated by higher-level medial frontal evaluative regions.

Anxiety

Rauch and colleagues used symptom provocation paradigms to study brain regions associated with symptoms in OCD (Rauch et al. 1994), SP (Rauch et al. 1995), and PTSD (Rauch et al. 1996) using $C^{15}O_2$ PET. In addition to analyzing results for individual diagnoses, data from these subject groups were pooled to determine the common mediating neuroanatomy of anxiety symptoms across these disorders (Rauch et al. 1997). Twenty right-handed subjects meeting clinical criteria for OCD ($n = 8$), SP ($n = 7$), or PTSD ($n = 8$) were studied during symptomatic and control conditions. Symptoms were provoked by stimuli individually tailored to each subject's clinical presentation, and control conditions were matched for sensorimotor and cognitive features (e.g., subjects with contamination obsessions were touched with a "contaminated" object during the provocation condition and with a "clean" version of the same object during the control condition).

Using SPM analysis, foci of significant activation in the provoked minus control state across the disorders were detected in right inferior frontal and posterior medial orbitofrontal cortex, and bilateral insular cortex, lenticulate nuclei, and brain stem. These results were noted to converge with those of a study of nonpathological anxiety, to reflect a possible role for paralimbic structures in a core neural system that mediates anxiety, and to support models of right-sided dominance in mediating emotional functions (at least in the case of negative valence). A statistically significant positive correlation was found between regional cerebral blood flow at the left brain stem focus and self-report anxiety scores, providing an "intriguing, but inconclusive glimpse regarding the role of human brain stem nuclei in mediating arousal or anxiety" (Rauch et al. 1997, p. 451).

Implications

The functional neuroimaging studies presented above suggest that symptoms of psychiatric disorders, such as those of neurologic disorders, can be localized to specific, phenomenologically relevant brain regions or circuits, despite an absence of gross brain pathology. Their results accord with those from other imaging studies, which reveal that similar neuropsychiatric symptoms—such as psychomotor poverty in schizophrenia and psychomotor retardation in depression—are associated with similar profiles of cerebral activity, regardless of diagnosis (Dolan et al. 1993). These observations suggest that neuropsychiatric disorders of diverse etiology could cause a similar symptom by affecting a particular final common neuroanatomical pathway, much the same way as a cerebral stroke, tumor, or abscess can all cause contralateral hemiparesis if they involve a motor pathway. Furthermore, the particular expression of the symptom could indicate the specific node or nodes in the distributed system/circuit that are affected or disconnected, much as pyramidal and extrapyramidal movement disorders or cortical and subcortical aphasias can now be discriminated (Damasio et al. 1982).

This model is supported by the convergence of clinical lesion, structural imaging, electrophysiologic, and functional imaging studies that suggest similar localizations for particular neurobehavioral symptoms, whether due to "idiopathic" psychiatric disorders or to known neurologic conditions. For example, left mesotemporal dysfunction has been implicated in the pathogenesis of psychosis, both by functional neuroimaging studies of schizophrenia (Liddle et al. 1992) and by the clinical and electrophysiological characterization of subjects with partial complex seizure disorders (Trimble 1991). Similarly, depression has been associated with left frontal strokes in structural MRI studies (Starkstein et al. 1987) and with left frontal hypoactivity on PET studies of subjects with primary major depression (Bench et al. 1993) or with depression secondary to movement disorders (Mayberg 1994). Furthermore, specific psychomotor and cognitive subsyndromes within the depressive spectrum have been associated with dysfunction in dorsolateral and medial prefrontal regions, respectively (Bench et al. 1993). Recently, a convergence of functional and structural changes in subgenual (medial) prefrontal cortex, as well as their possible relation to abnormal modulation of emotional processing in the amygdala and to state-dependent symptomatology, have been noted (Drevets 1999; Drevets et al. 1997).

CONCLUSION

In this chapter, we attempted to illustrate how, in the context of basic and clinical behavioral neuroscientific findings from related fields and convergent non-symptom-oriented techniques, functional neuroimaging studies with a focus on symptoms may engender a neuroanatomically/ functionally based understanding of neuropsychiatric disorders with implications for taxonomy, diagnosis, and treatment. Indeed, the latter has already begun to occur. In a functional neuroimaging study of subjects with unipolar depression, rostral anterior cingulate metabolism has been found to uniquely differentiate eventual serotonin-specific reuptake inhibitor (SSRI) responders from nonresponders (Mayberg 1997). Transcranial magnetic stimulation (TMS), a novel technique for altering cortical activity through application of a magnetic pulse, has been investigated in the treatment of persistent auditory hallucinations (Hoffman et al. 2000). Guided by the hallucinations study described above (Silbersweig et al. 1995), TMS (vs. sham stimulation) was administered to the left temporoparietal regions of 12 subjects with schizophrenia who have auditory hallucinations. This resulted in a significant reduction in hallucinations among the subjects. Similarly, investigations into the mechanism of action of psychotropic medications have increasingly focused on the specific cerebral regions modulated by relevant neurotransmitters. Neurochemical imaging studies using PET and single photon emission computed tomography (SPECT), sometimes combined with pharmacologic challenges, can provide an anatomically and clinically specific tool to accomplish this integration (Bremner et al. 2000; Drevets et al. 1999; Laruelle and Abi-Dargham 1999).

This evolving neurobiological understanding does not supplant previous phenomenologic approaches to psychiatric taxonomy. Indeed, just as Charcot's delineation of the signs and symptoms of Parkinson's disease laid the groundwork for an eventual identification of its pathophysiologic basis in the nigrostriatal system (Finger 2000), so the precise clinical descriptions of symptoms, syndromes, and mental functions provided by biological, descriptive, and dynamic psychiatrists are the bedrock upon which the neurobiological approach, including functional neuroimaging, rests. At the same time, this latter approach, informed by the burgeoning literature in the basic and cognitive neurosciences, may be able to elucidate previously unknown distinctions between, commonalities among, and mechanisms underlying psychiatric disorders, improving our ability both to diagnose and treat these prevalent and devastating conditions.

REFERENCES

American Psychiatric Association: Diagnostic and Statistical Manual of Mental Disorders, 4th Edition (DSM-IV). Washington, DC, American Psychiatric Association, 1994

Arana GW, Hyman SE: Handbook of Psychiatric Drug Therapy. Boston, Little, Brown and Company, 1991

Bench CJ, Friston KJ, Brown RG, et al: Regional cerebral blood flow in depression measured by positron emission tomography: the relationship with clinical dimensions. Psychol Med 23(3):579–590, 1993

Blumberg HP, Stern E, Martinez D, et al: Increased anterior cingulate and caudate activity in bipolar mania. Biol Psychiatry 48:1045–1052, 2000

Blumberg HP, Stern E, Ricketts S, et al: Rostral and orbital prefrontal cortex dysfunction in the manic state of bipolar disorder. Am J Psychiatry 156(12):1986–1988, 1999

Bremner JD, Innis RB, White T, et al: SPECT [I-123]iomazenil measurement of the benzodiazepine receptor in panic disorder. Biol Psychiatry 47(2):96–106, 2000

Buchel C, Coull JT, Friston KJ: The predictive value of changes in effective connectivity for human learning. Science 283(5407):1538–1541, 1999

Damasio AR, Damasio H, Rizzo M, et al: Aphasia with nonhemorrhagic lesions in the basal ganglia and internal capsule. Arch Neurol 39(1):15–24, 1982

Dolan RJ, Bench CJ, Liddle PF, et al: Dorsolateral prefrontal cortex dysfunction in the major psychoses: symptom or disease specificity? J Neurol Neurosurg Psychiatry 56(12):1290–1294, 1993

Drevets WC: Prefrontal cortical-amygdalar metabolism in major depression. Ann N Y Acad Sci 877:614–637, 1999

Drevets WC, Price JL, Simpson JR Jr, et al: Subgenual prefrontal cortex abnormalities in mood disorders. Nature 386(6627):824–827, 1997

Drevets WC, Frank E, Price JC, et al: PET imaging of serotonin 1A receptor binding in depression. Biol Psychiatry 46(10):1375–1387, 1999

Epstein J, Stern E, Silbersweig D: Mesolimbic activity associated with psychosis in schizophrenia: symptom-specific PET studies, in Advancing From the Ventral Striatum to the Extended Amygdala: Implications for Neuropsychiatry and Drug Abuse, Vol 877. Edited by McGinty JF. New York, New York Academy of Sciences, 1999, pp 562–574

Epstein J, Stern E, Silbersweig D: Neuropsychiatry at the millenium: the potential for mind/brain integration through emerging interdisciplinary research strategies. Clinical Neuroscience Research 1:10–18, 2001

Finger S: Minds Behind the Brain. New York, Oxford University Press, 2000

Finger S: Origins of Neuroscience: A History of Explorations Into Brain Function. New York, Oxford University Press, 1994

Fox PT, Raichle ME: Focal physiological uncoupling of cerebral blood flow and oxidative metabolism during somatosensory stimulation in human subjects. Proc Natl Acad Sci U S A 83(4):1140–1144, 1986

Friston KJ, Holmes AP, Worsley KJ, et al: Statistical parametric maps in functional imaging: a general linear approach. Human Brain Mapp 2(4):189–210, 1995

Grasby PM, Frith CD, Friston KJ, et al: A graded task approach to the functional mapping of brain areas implicated in auditory-verbal memory. Brain 117(Pt 6):1271–1282, 1994

Hoffman RE, Boutros NN, Hu S, et al: Transcranial magnetic stimulation and auditory hallucinations in schizophrenia (letter). Lancet 355(9209):1073–1075, 2000

Kandel ER: A new intellectual framework for psychiatry. Am J Psychiatry 155(4):457–469, 1998

Kwong KK, Belliveau JW, Chesler DA, et al: Dynamic magnetic resonance imaging of human brain activity during primary sensory stimulation. Proc Natl Acad Sci U S A 89(12):5675–5679, 1992

Laruelle M, Abi-Dargham A: Dopamine as the wind of the psychotic fire: new evidence from brain imaging studies. J Psychopharmacol 13(4):358–371, 1999

Liddle PF, Friston KJ, Frith CD, et al: Patterns of cerebral blood flow in schizophrenia. Br J Psychiatry 160:179–186, 1992

Llinas RR, Pare D: Of dreaming and wakefulness. Neuroscience 44(3):521–535, 1991

Manford M, Andermann F: Complex visual hallucinations. Clinical and neurobiological insights. Brain 121(Pt 10):1819–1840, 1998

Mayberg HS: Frontal lobe dysfunction in secondary depression. J Neuropsychiatry Clin Neurosci 6(4):428–442, 1994

Mayberg HS: Cingulate function in depression: a potential predictor of treatment response. Neuroreport 8:1057–1061, 1997

Mazziotta JC, Toga AW, Evans A, et al: A probabilistic atlas of the human brain: theory and rationale for its development. The International Consortium for Brain Mapping (ICBM). Neuroimage 2(2):89–101, 1995

McIntosh AR, Gonzalez-Lima F: Structural equation modeling and its application to network analysis in functional brain imaging. Human Brain Mapp 2:2–22, 1994

Ogawa S, Tank DW, Menon R, et al: Intrinsic signal changes accompanying sensory stimulation: functional brain mapping with magnetic resonance imaging. Proc Natl Acad Sci U S A 89(13):5951–5955, 1992

Ogawa S, Menon RS, Tank DW, et al: Functional brain mapping by blood oxygenation level-dependent contrast magnetic resonance imaging. A comparison of signal characteristics with a biophysical model. Biophys J 64(3):803–812, 1993

Posner MI, Petersen SE, Fox PT, et al: Localization of cognitive operations in the human brain. Science 240:1627–1631, 1988

Raichle, ME: Circulatory and metabolic correlates of brain function in normal humans, in Handbook of Physiology. V: The Nervous System. Edited by Mountcastle VB. Bethesda, MD, American Physiological Society, 1987, pp. 643–674

Rauch SL, Jenike MA, Alpert NM, et al: Regional cerebral blood flow measured during symptom provocation in obsessive-compulsive disorder using oxygen 15-labeled carbon dioxide and positron emission tomography. Arch Gen Psychiatry 51(1):62–70, 1994

Rauch SL, Savage CR, Alpert NM, et al: A positron emission tomographic study of simple phobic symptom provocation. Arch Gen Psychiatry 52(1):20–28, 1995

Rauch SL, van der Kolk BA, Fisler RE, et al: A symptom provocation study of post-traumatic stress disorder using positron emission tomography and script-driven imagery. Arch Gen Psychiatry 53(5):380–387, 1996

Rauch SL, Savage CR, Alpert NM, et al: The functional neuroanatomy of anxiety: a study of three disorders using positron emission tomography and symptom provocation. Biol Psychiatry 42(6):446–452, 1997

Rosen BR, Buckner RL, Dale AM: Event-related functional MRI: past, present, and future. Proc Natl Acad Sci U S A 95(3):773–780, 1998

Silbersweig DA, Stern E, Schnorr L, et al: Imaging transient, randomly occurring neuropsychological events in single subjects with positron emission tomography: an event-related count rate correlational analysis. J Cereb Blood Flow Metab 14(5):771–782, 1994

Silbersweig DA, Stern E, Frith C, et al: A functional neuroanatomy of hallucinations in schizophrenia. Nature 378(6553):176–179, 1995

Starkstein SE, Robinson RG, Price TR: Comparison of cortical and subcortical lesions in the production of poststroke mood disorders. Brain 110(Pt 4):1045–1059, 1987

Stern E, Silbersweig DA: Symptom capture: a strategy for pathophysiologic investigation in functional neuropsychiatric imaging, in Psychiatric Neuroimaging Research: Contemporary Strategies. Edited by Dougherty D, Rauch S. Washington, DC, American Psychiatric Publishing, 2001, pp 125–142

Stern E, Silbersweig DA, Chee KY, et al: A functional neuroanatomy of tics in Tourette syndrome. Arch Gen Psychiatry 57(8):741–748, 2000

Trimble MR: The Psychoses of Epilepsy. New York, Raven, 1991

Wong EC, Buxton RB, Frank LR: Quantitative perfusion imaging using arterial spin labeling. Neuroimaging Clin N Am 9(2):333–342, 1999

Worsley KJ, Friston KJ: Analysis of fMRI time-series revisited—again. Neuroimage 2(3):173–181, 1995

Yang YH, Frank JA, Hou L, et al: Multislice imaging of quantitative cerebral perfusion with pulsed arterial spin labeling. Magn Reson Med 39(5):825–832, 1998

6

Neuroimaging Studies of Mood Disorders

Wayne C. Drevets, M.D.

Neuroimaging technology provides unprecedented opportunities for elucidating the neurobiological correlates of mood disorders. Functional imaging tools such as positron emission tomography (PET), single photon emission computed tomography (SPECT), and functional magnetic resonance imaging (fMRI) have enabled in vivo characterization of neurophysiology in normal and pathological emotional states. Neurochemical imaging techniques using PET, SPECT, and magnetic resonance spectroscopy (MRS) provide in vivo quantitative analysis of neuroreceptor pharmacology, dynamic neurotransmitter function, and molecular biology. Structural magnetic resonance imaging (MRI) permits assessment of regional morphology and morphometry in primary psychiatric disorders and localization of pathology in psychiatric syndromes arising secondary to brain lesions.

The information gained about systems neuroanatomy through neuroimaging techniques becomes most useful when it is informed by data acquired using other experimental approaches. For example, in vivo neuroimaging data have begun to guide postmortem studies to discover neuropathological abnormalities in primary mood disorders. In the future, neuroimaging studies may also illuminate the etiology of psychiatric disorders by correlation of neuroimaging and genetic assessments.

This chapter reviews functional imaging data from depressed samples and integrates this information with findings from electrophysiological, lesion analysis, and histopathological studies to develop hypotheses about the pathobiology of mood disorders. Because the depression imaging literature is dominated by studies of resting neurophysiology [measured in terms of resting cerebral blood flow (CBF) or glucose metabolism], the findings from these studies are emphasized. The data that delineate brain regions where *function* is abnormal in mood disorders are discussed within the context of evidence from anatomical MRI and postmortem neuropathological studies showing areas where *structure* is also abnormal in these illnesses.

USE OF NEUROIMAGING TO INVESTIGATE DEPRESSION'S FUNCTIONAL ANATOMY

Interpretation of Differences in CBF and Metabolism Between Depressed Subjects and Control Subjects

The interpretation of neurophysiological differences between depressed and control subjects is complex. Because neural activity, CBF, and glucose metabolism are coupled, physiological images dynamically represent the functional anatomical correlates of cognitive, behavioral, or emotional processing in terms of changes in local hemodynamic function and metabolism. These changes reflect a summation of the chemical processes involved in neural activity, which is dominated by the energy utilization required to support terminal field synaptic transmission (DiRocco et al. 1989; Magistretti et al. 1995; Raichle 1987). Thus, local elevations of CBF and glucose metabolism signify increasing afferent synaptic transmission from local or distal structures in the experimental condition relative to the control condition, whereas reductions in these parameters reflect decreasing afferent transmission (DiRocco et al. 1989; Raichle 1987). Nevertheless, CBF and metabolism are also affected by neurotransmitter/receptor function, pathological alterations in the number of cells and/or synaptic contacts, and disease processes affecting cerebrovascular or thyroid function (Chimowitz et al. 1992; Drevets et al. 1999b; Fazekas 1989; Wooten and Collins 1981).

PET studies have identified neurophysiological abnormalities in multiple areas of the orbital and medial prefrontal cortex (PFC), amygdala, and related parts of the striatum and thalamus during the depressed phase of primary major depressive disorder (MDD) and bipolar disorder (BD; Figures 6-1 through 6-4). Some of these abnormalities appear mood state–dependent and are located in regions where CBF increases during normal and pathological emotional states. These differences between depressed

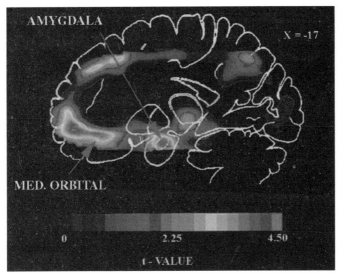

FIGURE 6-1 Areas of abnormally increased blood flow in FPDD shown in an image of t-values, produced by a voxel-by-voxel computation of the unpaired t-statistic to compare cerebral blood flow (CBF) between depressed subjects and control subjects (Drevets et al. 1992). The positive t-values in this sagittal section (x = −17 indicates 17 mm left of midline) show areas of increased CBF in the amygdala and medial (MED) orbital cortex of the depressed subjects. Abnormal activity in these regions in major depressive disorder was confirmed using higher resolution, glucose metabolic measures in other studies. Anterior is to the left. (Figure is available in color in original source.)

Source. Adapted from Price JL, Carmichael ST, Drevets WC: "Networks Related to the Orbital and Medial Prefrontal Cortex: A Substrate for Emotional Behavior?" *Prog Brain Res* 107:523–536, 1996, with permission from Elsevier Science.

and control subjects may thus implicate areas where physiological activity changes to mediate or respond to the emotional, behavioral, and cognitive manifestations of major depressive episodes (MDE). Other abnormalities persist following symptom remission and are found in orbital and medial PFC areas where postmortem studies demonstrate reductions in cortex volume and histopathological changes in primary mood disorders. Evidence from brain mapping, lesion analysis, and electrophysiological studies of humans and/or experimental animals suggests these areas participate in modulating emotional behavior and stress responses. Dysfunction involving these regions may thus play a role in the pathogenesis of depressive symptoms.

Mood state–dependent *decreases* in CBF and metabolism are also found during MDE in areas implicated in attentional, visuospatial, and sensory processing (reviewed in Drevets and Raichle 1998). Interpreting these

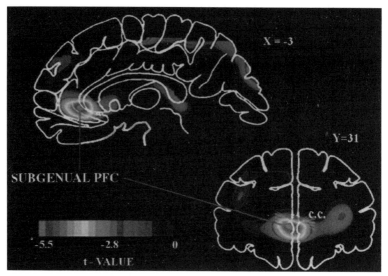

FIGURE 6-2 Coronal (y = 31 indicates 31 mm anterior to the anterior commissure) and sagittal (3 mm left of midline, or x = −3) sections, showing negative voxel t-values where glucose metabolism is *decreased* in depressed subjects relative to control subjects (Drevets et al. 1997). The reduction in metabolism in this region appeared to be accounted for by a corresponding reduction in cortex volume. Although none of these subjects were involved in the study that generated the t-image shown in Figure 6-1, the mean metabolism in this independent set of depressed subjects was also abnormally *increased* in the amygdala and orbital cortex. Anterior is to the left. (Figure is available in color in original source.)
Source. Reprinted with permission from Drevets WC, Price JL, Simpson JR, et al.: "Subgenual Prefrontal Cortex Abnormalities in Mood Disorders." *Nature* 386:824–827, 1997. Copyright 1997 Macmillan Magazines Limited.

observations requires an understanding of the regulation of neurophysiological activity across anatomical systems. Brain mapping studies show that while CBF increases in brain regions putatively activated to perform an experimental task, CBF concomitantly *decreases* in some other neural systems that appear *nonessential* to task performance (Drevets and Raichle 1998). Such "deactivated" areas are believed to reflect attention-related processes whereby signal processing is enhanced via suppression of neural transmission conveying competing, unattended information (Drevets et al. 1995a; Posner and Presti 1987; Whang et al. 1991). These phenomena are exemplified by the patterns of reduced CBF seen during expectation of somatosensory stimuli. In these patterns, CBF decreases in the human first (SI) and second somatosensory cortex located outside the cortical representation of the skin area targeted by an expected stimulus; however, CBF does not change in the somatosensory cortex representing the skin locus of the awaited stimulation (Drevets et al. 1995a). These results concur with electrophysiological evidence of suppression, or "gating," of

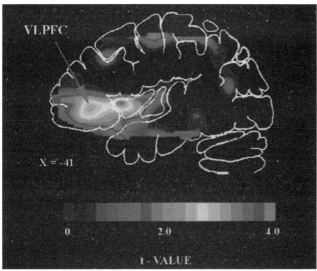

FIGURE 6-3   Sagittal t-image section 41 mm left of midline (X = −41), showing an area of increased cerebral blood flow in depressed subjects relative to control subjects in the left ventrolateral prefrontal cortex (VLPFC), lateral orbital cortex, and anterior insula (Drevets et al. 1992). (Figure is available in color in original source.)
Source. Reprinted from Drevets WC: "Functional Neuroimaging Studies of Depression: The Anatomy of Melancholia." *Annu Rev Med* 49:341–361, 1998. Used with permission.

sensory input to SI cortical neurons when the cutaneous receptive field of the recorded cell is not engaged during tactile discrimination behavior and preserved to fields where behaviorally significant stimuli are expected (Chapin and Woodward 1982; Chapman and Ageranioti-Bélanger 1991). In PET images, the reduction of CBF in portions of SI representing unattended skin sites is presumably accounted for by reduced afferent synaptic transmission into these areas (DiRocco et al. 1989; Drevets et al. 1995a). Similar interactions also occur across sensory modalities (reviewed in Drevets and Raichle 1998). For example, CBF decreases in primary auditory cortex, auditory association cortex, somatosensory cortex, and posterior cingulate cortex as subjects process complex visual stimuli (Haxby et al. 1994).

Areas specialized for emotional versus higher cognitive functions also appear to engage in such cross-modal relationships. In amygdalar, posterior orbital cortex, and ventromedial PFC sites where CBF increases during emotion-related tasks, flow *decreases* during performance of attentionally demanding, cognitive tasks (Drevets and Raichle 1998; Shulman et al. 1997). Conversely, in dorsal anterior cingulate and dorsolateral prefrontal cortex (DLPFC) areas where flow increases while performing attentionally

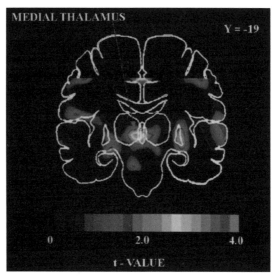

FIGURE 6-4 Coronal t-image section 19 mm posterior to the anterior commissure (Y = −19), showing the area of increased cerebral blood flow in the left medial thalamus of depressed subjects relative to control subjects (Drevets et al. 1992, 1995b). (Figure is available in color in original source.)

Source. Reprinted from Drevets WC: "Functional Neuroimaging Studies of Depression: The Anatomy of Melancholia." *Annu Rev Med* 49:341–361, 1998. Used with permission.

demanding cognitive tasks, flow *decreases* during some emotional states (Drevets and Raichle 1998; Mayberg et al. 1999).

These reciprocal patterns of neural activity hold intriguing implications for interactions between emotion and cognition (Drevets and Raichle 1998). During depression, the reduction of CBF in dorsal anterior cingulate and DLPFC areas specialized for verbal, attentional, visuospatial, and mnemonic processing may reflect suppression of afferent neural transmission while dysphoric emotions or thoughts are processed. This phenomenon may conceivably relate to the subtle impairments of attention, memory, and visuospatial function that may be associated with MDE (Drevets and Raichle 1998).

Critical Assessment of the Psychiatric Imaging Literature

The literature is in disagreement regarding the specific locations and direction of neurophysiological abnormalities in MDD. Many inconsistencies across studies may be resolved by critical assessment of experimental design and data analysis (Drevets and Botteron 1997; Raichle 1987). The sensitivity for identifying abnormalities in psychiatric imaging studies is affected by sample size, medication effects, technical limitations of imaging acquisition and analysis, and biological heterogeneity within mood-disordered samples. Issues related to subject selection, image acquisition, and image analysis that are particularly relevant for interpreting studies of depression are briefly reviewed here.

Technical Issues of Image Acquisition

Although glucose metabolism is typically measured using PET and [^{18}F]fluorodeoxyglucose (FDG), CBF can be measured using PET and $H_2{}^{15}O$, SPECT or non-tomographic multidetector systems and ^{133}Xe, or SPECT and ^{123}I-labeled or ^{99m}technician-labeled lipophilic agents (e.g., ^{123}I-iodoamphetamine and ^{99m}Tc-HMPAO [Raichle 1987] methods for quantitating absolute CBF using MRI are also under development). Some of these methods have limitations that must be considered in reviewing the depression imaging literature. For example, the photon emitted by the decay of ^{133}Xe is characterized by relatively low energy, so CBF measures acquired using this method are limited to the cortical gray matter lying within approximately 2 cm of the scalp, precluding assessment of limbic, basal ganglia, and basal/medial frontal and temporal lobe structures (Raichle 1987). In addition, perfusion measures using ^{123}I-iodoamphetamine and ^{99m}Tc-HMPAO have the limitation that *measured* blood flow falls off the "line of identity" with *actual* blood flow at the upper end of the physiological range. Thus, although measured perfusion correlates well with CBF in conditions associated with reduced flow (e.g., cerebrovascular disease), the sensitivity for detecting changes in CBF is relatively low in conditions in which CBF increases (e.g., neural activation during sensory stimulation of neuropsychological task performance). Finally, because CBF is not easily quantitated using these SPECT tracers, many studies have normalized regional perfusion data by cerebellar perfusion.

This approach has been an important error source among SPECT studies of depression because PET studies have shown that cerebellar flow increases during depressive and anxious states (e.g., Bench et al. 1992; Drevets and Botteron 1997). Perfusion in other structures may therefore appear artifactually decreased in depressed relative to control subjects when normalized to cerebellar flow. This problem is evident in SPECT studies, which report perfusion ratios normalized to other control regions of interest (ROI) or provide whole cortex-to-perfusion ratios to aid in interpreting regional-to-cerebellar ratio. Although these studies reported that frontal and temporal cortex perfusion is decreased in MDD when expressed as a regional-to-cerebellar ratio, these abnormalities largely or completely disappear when expressed instead as regional-to-occipital (Philpot et al. 1993) or regional-to-whole cortex (Mayberg et al. 1994) perfusion ratios.

Technical Issues Involved in Image Analysis

The neuroimaging abnormalities found in MDD have been subtle relative to the variability of imaging measures, with effect sizes generally less than two and often less than one. As a result, the abnormalities associated with psychiatric illness cannot be detected using the traditional radiological approach of simple image inspection and are instead identified as quantitative differences between the mean values of ill and control samples. To compare image data across groups, regional radiotracer concentration is sampled using either ROI or voxel-by-voxel analyses. Each method requires trade-offs between Type I and Type II error, which affect the sensitivity for detecting differences between depressed and control subjects (Drevets 2000; Poline et al. 1997).

State-of-the-art ROI approaches involve circumscribing volumes of interest in anatomical MRI images that have been coregistered to the same subject's PET image, so the PET measures can be precisely localized (Woods et al. 1993). This approach provides the greatest sensitivity for detecting abnormalities when an affected region can be delimited in MRI scans. However, ROI placement may undersample or dilute focal abnormalities when anatomical boundaries are unknown.

To address these Type II error sources, statistical parametric mapping techniques are used to survey brain images voxel by voxel to reveal inherent differences between groups or conditions (e.g., Figures 6-1 through 6-4; Drevets et al. 1992; Friston et al. 1991). Primary tomographs are spatially transformed into a standardized stereotaxic space so image data can be averaged across subjects. Because current spatial transformation algorithms do not precisely align the variable, complex, three-dimensional (3-D) structure of images from different brains, images are blurred ("filtered") prior to analysis to reduce the effects of misalignment error (Poline et al. 1997). The resulting loss of spatial resolution from blurring and the error in overlaying brain structure across subjects decrease sensitivity for detecting abnormalities in small structures (e.g., subgenual PFC, amygdala) or areas characterized by high anatomical variability (e.g., orbital cortex).

Voxel-by-voxel analyses also increase Type I error because they require tens of thousands of statistical comparisons. This problem can be dealt with by correcting P values for the number of independent resolution elements in the search area (Poline et al. 1997). Alternatively, the area where voxel-by-voxel analysis reveals inherent differences between groups can be used to guide ROI placement and the statistical significance of an intergroup difference established by replication within this ROI in an independent subject sample (Drevets et al. 1992, 1995c, 1997). Unfortunately, few published studies of depression have been appropriately corrected for the number of comparisons, so the literature is filled with reports of "abnormalities" that cannot be distinguished from multiple-comparison artifact.

Design Issues Involved in Sample Selection

Antidepressant, antianxiety, or antipsychotic drug treatments can decrease CBF and metabolism in frontal, parietal, and temporal lobe regions (reviewed in Drevets et al. 1999b). Studies including images from subjects taking such agents usually fail to detect the areas of hypermetabolism identified in unmedicated depressed subjects and instead report areas of reduced CBF or metabolism not evident in unmedicated samples. Nevertheless, only a minority of studies imaged subjects in an unmedicated state.

A Type II error source that presents a greater challenge for the design of imaging studies is the clinical and biological heterogeneity extant within subject samples meeting criteria for MDD. Some of the variability seen in imaging studies of mood disorders may be accounted for by clinical differences in severity, chronicity, or signs/symptoms (e.g., psychomotor retardation/agitation). Variability may also stem from the likelihood that the diagnostic criteria for MDD and BD encompass groups of disorders that are heterogeneous with respect to etiology and pathophysiology (Drevets and Todd 1997; Winokur 1997).

In some studies, selecting subjects with familial mood disorders reduced variability. Subjects with primary, familial MDD [i.e., familial pure depressive disease (FPDD)] were previously shown to be more likely to have abnormalities of hypothalamic-pituitary-adrenal (HPA) axis function, platelet [^{3}H]-imipramine binding, and sleep electroencephalogram (EEG) relative to MDD subjects who either lacked mood-disordered relatives or had first-degree relatives with alcoholism or antisocial personality disorder (Kupfer et al. 1992; Lewis and McChesney 1985; Winokur 1982, 1997). Depressed samples with FPDD or BD have also been more likely to show elevated CBF and metabolism in the amygdala, orbital cortex, and medial thalamus, and decreased metabolism and cortex volume in the subgenual PFC than nonfamilial cases or cases whose depressive syndromes arose secondary to other medical/psychiatric conditions (Drevets et al. 1992, 1995b, 1997, 1999b; Hirayasu et al. 1999; Kegeles et al. 1999; Öngür et al. 1998). However, studies using alternative means for selecting enriched MDD samples, such as melancholic subtype criteria or responsiveness to sleep deprivation or phototherapy, have also found elevated metabolism in the amygdala and orbital cortex during MDE (Cohen et al. 1992; Ebert et al. 1991; Nofzinger et al. 1999; Wu et al. 1992).

The mood-disordered subtype for which a distinct set of neuroimaging findings has been best characterized is composed of elderly depressed subjects with a late age at illness onset. Depressed subjects with onset of first MDE after age 55 are more likely than both age-matched, healthy control subjects and age-matched depressed subjects with an earlier age at onset to have large "patches" of magnetic resonance (MR) signal hyperintensity (in T2 weighted images) in the deep and periventricular white matter and lacunae in the cortex and striatum (Drevets et al. 1999b; Krishnan et al. 1993). Tissue acquired postmortem from brain areas showing patches of MR signal hyperintensity reveals arteriosclerosis, gliosis, white matter necrosis, and axon loss within the affected areas but not in surrounding tissue where the MRI signal appears normal (Awad et al. 1986; Chimowitz et al. 1992). Functional imaging studies confirm that CBF is decreased in areas where white matter hyperintensities (WMH) are evident in MR images (Chimowitz et al. 1992; Fazekas 1989). Subjects with late onset of depression also commonly have enlarged cerebral ventricles, widened cortical sulci, and reduced frontal lobe and basal ganglia volumes that are believed to reflect tissue atrophy secondary to ischemia (reviewed in Drevets et al. 1999b). Because cerebrovascular disease alters radiotracer delivery, metabolic activity, and relationships between neuronal activity, CBF, and oxygen extraction (Deryden et al. 1998), the functional imaging correlates of subjects with late-onset MDD differ from those of depressed subjects with early- or midlife-onset of illness (Drevets et al. 1999b). Nevertheless, most imaging studies of MDD that included elderly subjects failed to distinguish or exclude such subjects, confounding interpretation of their results.

The MRI and clinical correlates of late-onset depression are hypothesized to indicate that this mood-disordered subgroup develops MDE secondary to cerebrovascular disease (Krishnan et al. 1993). The left frontal lobe and striatum are the regions most commonly affected by WMH or lacunae in late-onset MDD. These are the same regions where infarction increases the risk for developing MDE following stroke (reviewed in Drevets et al. 1999b; Starkstein and Robinson 1989). These regions also contain neuropathological abnormalities that are of a distinct, idiopathic nature (see below) in familial MDD and BD subjects studied early in life. Thus, dysfunction involving the same brain structures may confer vulnerability to MDE in both early- and late-onset mood disorders.

However, abnormalities in other brain systems may be specific to particular mood disorder subgroups. For example, serotonin$_{1A}$ receptor imaging studies using PET and [*carbonyl*-^{11}C]WAY100635 (Drevets et al. 1999a; Sargent et al. 2000) converge with in vitro studies acquired postmortem (Bowen et al. 1989; López et al. 1998) or antemortem (Francis et al. 1989) to indicate that 5-HT$_{1A}$ receptor binding is abnormally decreased in primary

MDD and BD. In contrast, the results of studies of suicide victims who may have secondary mood disorders or neuropsychiatric conditions other than mood disorders have been highly variable (reviewed in Drevets et al. 1999b).

FUNCTIONAL ANATOMICAL CORRELATES OF MAJOR DEPRESSION

Many of the brain regions where neuroimaging studies show physiological and anatomical abnormalities in MDD and BD participate in the neural circuitry underlying the modulation and expression of emotional behavior. The neuroimaging findings in these regions in depression and the information available regarding these structures' function in emotional behavior are reviewed in the following sections.

Subgenual Anterior Cingulate Cortex

The anterior cingulate cortex situated anterior and ventral to the genu of the corpus callosum [termed "pregenual" (Drevets et al. 1992) and "subgenual" (Drevets et al. 1997), respectively] have been implicated by numerous studies of MDD and BD (reviewed in Drevets and Raichle 1998; Drevets 1999). In the subgenual PFC, CBF and metabolism are decreased in unipolar and bipolar depressed subjects relative to healthy control subjects (Figure 6-2; Buchsbaum et al. 1997; Drevets et al. 1997; Kegeles et al. 1999). This abnormality appears to be accounted for by a left-lateralized, volumetric reduction of the corresponding cortex, initially demonstrated by MRI-based morphometric measures (Drevets et al. 1997) and later by postmortem neuropathological studies of familial BD and MDD (Öngür et al. 1998). This reduction in volume exists early in the illness in familial BD (Hirayasu et al. 1999) and MDD (Botteron et al., in press); however, preliminary evidence from one study of twins discordant for MDD suggests that it follows illness onset (Botteron et al. 1999). Although effective treatment with selective serotonin reuptake inhibitor (SSRI) antidepressant drugs did not alter subgenual PFC volume in MDD subjects (Drevets et al. 1997), this measure was significantly increased in BD subjects who were chronically medicated with lithium or divalproex relative to clinically similar subjects who were not medicated with these agents (Drevets et al., manuscript in preparation). Chronic administration of these mood stabilizers increases expression of the neurotrophic protein, Bcl-2, in the frontal cortex, striatum, and mesiotemporal of experimental animals (Manji et al. 1999). Bcl-2 increases neurite sprouting and protects against glutamate-mediated excitoxicity.

This raises the possibility that the difference in subgenual PFC volume in BD subjects treated with lithium or divalproex reflects a neuroprotective/neurotrophic effect of these medications (Manji et al. 1999).

Baseline CBF and metabolism appear abnormally decreased in PET images during MDE; however, computer simulations that correct PET images for the partial volume effect expected from a reduction in gray matter volume indicate that the "actual" metabolic activity in the remaining subgenual PFC tissue is *increased* in depressed relative to control subjects. This hypothesis appears compatible with findings that effective antidepressant treatments *decrease* metabolic activity in this region in MDD (Buchsbaum et al. 1997; Drevets 1999; Mayberg et al. 1999). Computer simulations of *posttreatment* images find that actual (partial volume-corrected) metabolism decreases to normative levels during effective treatment. This mood state dependency of subgenual PFC metabolism would appear consistent with PET studies showing that flow increases in the subgenual PFC of healthy, nondepressed humans during experimentally induced sadness (Damasio et al. 1998; George et al. 1995; Mayberg et al. 1999).

The subgenual PFC is extensively and reciprocally interconnected to areas implicated in emotional behavior such as the posterior orbital cortex, hypothalamus, amygdala, accumbens, ventral tegmental area (VTA), raphe, locus coeruleus, periaqueductal gray (PAG), and nucleus tractus solitarius (Figure 6-5; Carmichael and Price 1995; Leichnetz and Astruc 1976). Humans with lesions that include subgenual PFC show abnormal autonomic responses to emotionally provocative stimuli, inability to experience emotion related to concepts that ordinarily evoke emotion, and inability to use information regarding the probability of punishment and reward in guiding social behavior (Damasio et al. 1990). In rats, bilateral or *right*-lateralized lesions of the prelimbic (the apparent homolog of primate subgenual PFC) and infralimbic cortices *attenuate* sympathetic autonomic responses, corticosterone secretion, and gastric stress pathology during restraint stress or exposure to fear-conditioned stimuli (Frysztak and Neafsey 1994; Morgan and LeDoux 1995; Sullivan and Gratton 1999). In contrast, *left*-sided lesions of this area *increase* sympathetic autonomic arousal and corticosterone responses to restraint stress (Sullivan and Gratton 1999). These data suggest that the right subgenual PFC facilitates expression of visceral responses during emotional processing, whereas the left subgenual PFC inhibits such responses (Sullivan and Gratton 1999).

If so, the left-lateralized volumetric reduction of the subgenual PFC in MDD and BD may contribute to the sympathetic autonomic arousal and heightened HPA axis activity seen in depression (Carney et al. 1988; Dioro et al. 1993; Holsboer 1995; Veith et al. 1994). HPA axis dysregulation in mood disorders has been believed to partly involve a disturbance of negative feedback inhibition of cortisol release at the level of the limbic system

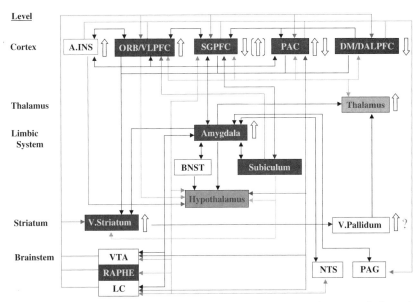

FIGURE 6-5 Anatomical circuits implicated by neuroimaging and neuropathological studies of mood disorders. The abnormalities summarized are hypothesized to contribute to the pathogenesis of disturbances of emotional processing. Regions in dark shading are reported to have volumetric and/or histopathological abnormalities in primary major depressive disorder and/or bipolar disorder (see text). Regions in light shading have not been microscopically examined in mood disorders but are areas where structural abnormalities are *suspected* based on the finding of third ventricle enlargement in children and adults with bipolar disorder. Open arrows to the right of each region indicate the direction of abnormalities in cerebral blood flow (CBF) and metabolism in depressed subjects versus control subjects (the ? indicates where experimental data await replication). Open arrows in parentheses indicate the direction of metabolic abnormalities after correcting PET measures for the partial volume effects of reduced gray matter volume [(?)-indicates where decreased gray matter is suspected as the explanation for reductions in CBF and metabolism, but partial volume–corrected PET results have not been reported]. Solid lines indicate major anatomical connections between structures, with closed arrowheads indicating the direction of the projecting axons (reciprocal connections have arrowheads at both ends). Affected prefrontal cortex (PFC) areas include the ventrolateral and orbital PFC (ORB/VLPFC), the anterior (agranular) insula (A.INS), the anterior cingulate gyrus ventral and anterior to the genu of the corpus callosum [subgenual PFC (SGPFC) and pregenual anterior cingulate (PAC), respectively], and the dorsomedial/dorsal anterolateral PFC (DM/DALPFC). The parts of the striatum under consideration are the ventromedial caudate and nucleus accumbens, which project to the ventral pallidum (Nauta and Domesick 1984). The major dopaminergic projections to these areas are from the ventral tegmental area (VTA). Other abbreviations: BNST = bed nucleus of the stria terminalis; LC = locus coeruleus; NTS = nucleus tractus solitarius; PAG = periaqueductal gray. (Figure is available in color in original source.)

Source. Reprinted from Drevets WC: "Neuroimaging and Neuropathological Studies of Depression: Implications for the Cognitive-Emotional Features of Mood Disorders." *Current Opinion on Neurobiology* 11:240–249, 2001; originally adapted and reprinted by permission of Elsevier Science from Drevets WC: "Neuroimaging Studies of Mood Disorders." *Biol Psychiatry* 48:813–829, 2000. Copyright 2000 by the Society of Biological Psychiatry.

(Holsboer 1995; Young et al. 1993). Stimulation of the glucocorticoid receptors situated in the ventral anterior cingulate area of the rat, which appears partly homologous to the human subgenual PFC, has been shown to inhibit stress-induced corticosterone release (Dioro et al. 1993). Furthermore, the hypothesis that left-sided, ventromedial PFC lesions disinhibit the facilitation of emotional expression mediated by the right ventromedial PFC (Sullivan and Grattan 1999) is noteworthy in light of PET data showing that *right* subgenual PFC metabolism correlates positively with depression severity in MDD (Drevets 2000).

Finally, the subgenual PFC may participate in evaluating the reward-related potential of stimuli or behavior by modulating mesolimbic dopaminergic function. The subgenual PFC sends efferent projections to the VTA and the substantia nigra (Leichnetz and Astruc 1976; Price 1999; Sesack and Pickel 1992), and is part of the anterior cingulate cortex area that receives particularly dense dopaminergic innervation from the VTA (Crino et al. 1993). In rats, electrical or glutamatergic stimulation of medial PFC areas that include prelimbic C elicits burst firing patterns from VTA dopaminergic cells and increases dopamine (DA) release in the accumbens (Murase et al. 1993; Taber and Fibiger 1993). Because the phasic, burst firing patterns of dopamine (DA) neurons appear to participate in encoding information regarding stimuli that predict reward, as well as deviations between such predictions and the actual occurrence of reward (Schultz 1997), it is conceivable that subgenual PFC dysfunction contributes to the disturbances of hedonic perception and motivated behavior seen in mood disorders (Fibiger 1991). In this regard, the magnitude of abnormal metabolic activity in the subgenual PFC may relate to switches between depression and mania, as subgenual PFC metabolism was markedly increased in small samples of manic subjects relative to both depressed and healthy control subjects (e.g., Drevets et al. 1997).

Pregenual Anterior Cingulate Cortex

The literature is less consistent with respect to the functional status of the pregenual anterior cingulate cortex. This region consistently shows elevated CBF during various emotional conditions elicited in healthy or anxiety-disordered humans (reviewed in Drevets and Raichle 1998). Electrical stimulation of this region elicits fear, panic, or a sense of foreboding in humans and vocalization in experimental animals (reviewed in Price et al. 1996).

Many imaging studies find that CBF and metabolism are increased in this area during MDE (reviewed in Drevets 1999). Mayberg et al. (1997)

more specifically reported that, although metabolism in this area was abnormally increased in depressed subjects who subsequently showed a good response to antidepressants, metabolism was abnormally decreased in depressed subjects who had poor or incomplete treatment responses. In contrast, other groups found inverse correlations between resting metabolism and subsequent antidepressant response in MDD, with lower baseline pregenual anterior cingulate metabolism predicting superior responsiveness to antidepressants (Brody et al. 1999a; Ketter et al. 1999). Treatment effects on pregenual anterior cingulate CBF and metabolism have also differed across studies, with activity decreasing in some but increasing in others in posttreatment relative to pretreatment scans (reviewed in Drevets 1999). The extent to which these discrepancies are explained by differential effects in subregions of the anterior cingulate remains unclear.

Amygdala

Resting CBF and glucose metabolism are abnormally elevated in the amygdala in MDD subjects with FPDD, Type II BD, or nonpsychotic Type I BD (Figures 6-1 and 6-6; Abercrombie et al. 1996; Drevets et al. 1992, 1995b; Wu et al. 1992). In contrast, this abnormality is not evident in more severe, psychotic BD Type I subjects (Drevets 1995) or MDD samples meeting Winokur (1982) criteria for depression spectrum disease (Drevets et al. 1995c). Abnormalities of resting amygdalar CBF/metabolism have also not been found in obsessive-compulsive disorder (OCD), panic disorder, phobic disorders, or schizophrenia, suggesting this abnormality may be specific to some primary mood disorder subtypes (reviewed in Drevets and Botteron 1997).

In subjects with FPDD, the magnitude of this abnormality as measured by PET is approximately 5% to 6% relative to healthy control subjects, which when corrected for the spatial resolution effects of PET images would reflect an actual increase in amygdala CBF and metabolism of 50% to 70% (Drevets et al. 1992; Links et al. 1996). These magnitudes are in the physiological range, as CBF measured by tissue autoradiography increases approximately 50% in the rat amygdala during exposure to fear-conditioned stimuli (LeDoux et al. 1983). The abnormal elevation in amygdala metabolism in major depression does not appear to be accounted for by a heightened stress response to scanning, because amygdala metabolism remains abnormally increased in MDD during sleep. Nofzinger et al. (1999) reported that, although amygdala metabolism is increased in depressed versus control subjects during wakefulness, the normal increase in metabolism that occurs during rapid eye movement (REM) sleep is also greater in depressed than in control subjects.

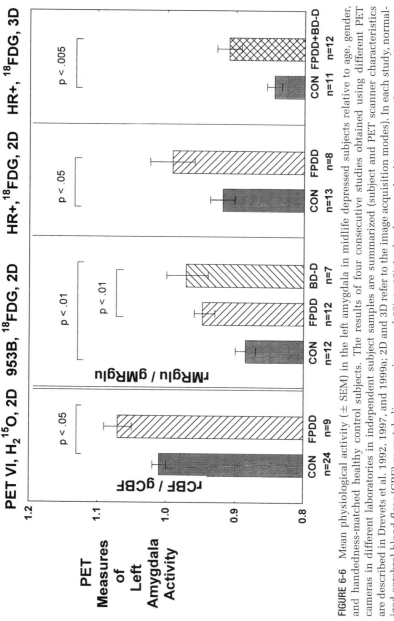

FIGURE 6-6   Mean physiological activity (± SEM) in the left amygdala in midlife depressed subjects relative to age, gender, and handedness-matched healthy control subjects. The results of four consecutive studies obtained using different PET cameras in different laboratories in independent subject samples are summarized (subject and PET scanner characteristics are described in Drevets et al. 1992, 1997, and 1999a; 2D and 3D refer to the image acquisition modes). In each study, normalized cerebral blood flow (CBF) or metabolism was increased 6% to 8% in the depressed subjects versus the control subjects (whole-brain CBF and metabolism did not significantly differ between depressed subjects and control subjects in these studies). *Abbreviations:* rCBF/gCBF = regional-to-global cerebral blood flow ratio; rMRglu/gMRglu = ratio of regional-to-global metabolic rates for glucose; CON = control subjects; FPDD = familial pure depressive disease (Winokur 1982); BD-D = depressed phase of bipolar disorder.

Amygdalar CBF and metabolism correlate positively with depression severity (Abercrombie et al. 1996; Drevets et al. 1992, 1995b). Nevertheless, CBF and metabolism in the left amygdala appear abnormally increased (although to a lesser extent) during the unmedicated, remitted phase of FPDD (i.e., between MDE; Drevets et al. 1992). Conversely, during antidepressant treatment that both induces and maintains symptom remission, amygdala metabolism decreases to normative levels, compatible with preclinical evidence that chronic antidepressant administration has inhibitory effects on amygdala function (reviewed in Drevets 1999). Moreover, antidepressant-medicated, remitted subjects with MDD who relapse in response to serotonin depletion (via tryptophan-free diet) have higher amygdala metabolism prior to depletion than similar subjects who do not relapse (Bremner et al. 1997). Abnormal amygdala activity may thus relate to the susceptibility to MDE recurrence, as well as to MDE severity.

The positive correlation between amygdala metabolism and depression severity rated by scales that assess diverse clinical signs and symptoms of MDE may reflect the amygdala's role in organizing multiple aspects of emotional/stress responses. Electrical stimulation of the amygdala in nondepressed humans can produce anxiety, fear, dysphoria, recollection of emotionally valenced events, and increased cortisol secretion (Brothers 1995; Gloor et al. 1982; Rubin et al. 1966). Depressive signs such as social withdrawal, inactivity, panic attacks, and reduced pain sensitivity may conceivably be explained by amygdalar stimulation of the PAG, because in experimental animals stimulation of ventrolateral PAG produces social withdrawal, behavioral quiescence, and hypoalgesia, whereas stimulation of lateral PAG produces defensive behaviors, sympathetic autonomic arousal, and hypoalgesia (reviewed in Price 1999). The elevated sympathetic tone (e.g., manifested by increased norepinephrine secretion and resting heart rate) and arousal seen in MDD could also reflect transmission of excessive amygdala activity via efferent projections to the lateral hypothalamus and locus coeruleus (Carney et al. 1988; Davis 1992; Veith et al. 1994). In addition, the amygdala facilitates stress-related corticotropin-releasing hormone (CRH) release via both intrinsic CRH containing neurons and bisynaptic (double GABA-ergic) anatomical projections to the paraventricular nucleus (Herman and Cullinan 1997), so excessive amygdala activity may play a role in CRH hypersecretion in mood disorders (Feldman et al. 1994; Musselman and Nemeroff 1993). Finally, activation of the amygdalar projections to the ventral striatum arrest goal-directed behavior in experimental animals (Mogenson et al. 1993), suggesting a possible neural mechanism for the cessation of reward-directed or motivated behavior during MDE.

Orbital Cortex

In the left and right posterior orbital cortex, the left ventrolateral PFC (VLPFC), as well as the anterior (agranular) insula, CBF, and metabolism, are abnormally *increased* in unmedicated subjects with primary MDD (Figures 6-1 and 6-3; e.g., Baxter et al. 1987 [see table 3 of this reference], Biver et al. 1994; Cohen et al. 1992; Drevets et al. 1992, 1995c; Ebert et al. 1991). Flow and metabolism also increase in these areas during experimentally induced sadness and anxiety in healthy subjects and during induced anxiety and obsessional states in subjects with OCD, posttraumatic stress disorder, simple phobic disorders, and panic disorders (reviewed in Drevets and Raichle 1998). The elevation of physiological activity in these areas during MDE appears mood state dependent, as a variety of effective, somatic antidepressant therapies result in decreases in CBF and metabolism in the remitted relative to the depressed phase of MDD (e.g., Brody et al. 1999; Drevets 1999; Drevets et al. 1992; Mayberg et al. 1999; Nobler et al. 1994).

A complex relationship exists between depression severity and metabolic activity in the orbital cortex and VLPFC. Although CBF and metabolism are elevated in these areas in depressed subjects relative to the remitted phase of MDD, these measures correlate inversely with ratings of depression severity and depressive ideation (Drevets et al. 1992, 1995c). Compatible with these data, although metabolic activity is abnormally increased in these areas in outpatient, treatment-responsive, unipolar and bipolar depressed subjects, more severely ill or treatment-refractory BD samples and inpatient MDD samples have shown mean CBF and metabolic values that either did not significantly differ or were decreased relative to control subjects (Drevets et al. 1997; Ketter et al. 1999; Mayberg et al. 1997).

These relationships between orbital metabolism and depression severity are consistent with evidence from imaging, lesion analysis, and electrophysiological studies that portions of this cortex participate in modulating behavioral and visceral responses associated with defensive, fear, and reward-directed behavior as reinforcement contingencies change. Posterior orbital cortex CBF also increases in subjects with OCD and animal phobia during exposure to phobic stimuli and in healthy subjects during induced sadness (Drevets et al. 1995b; Rauch et al. 1994; Schneider et al. 1995). In these cases, the change in posterior orbital cortex CBF correlates inversely with concomitant changes in obsessive thinking, anxiety, and sadness, respectively. In animal-phobic subjects, PET images acquired during repeated exposures to a phobic stimulus revealed that orbital flow was unchanged during initial exposures when the fear response was greatest but progressively increased as subjects habituated to the stimulus during subsequent exposures, with CBF correlating inversely with changes in anxiety ratings and heart rate (Drevets et al. 1995b).

Nearly one-half of pyramidal cells in the orbital cortex alter their firing rates during the delay period between stimulus and response, and patterns of posttrial activity—which relate to the presence or absence of reinforcement—suggest these cells play a role in extinguishing unreinforced responses to appetitive or aversive stimuli (Rolls 1995). This function appears to involve interactions with the amygdala and other limbic structures (Mogenson et al. 1993; Price et al. 1996). The orbital cortex and amygdala send direct projections to each other and overlapping projections to the striatum, hypothalamus, and PAG, through which they modulate each other's transmission (Figure 6-5; Carmichael and Price 1995; Garcia et al. 1999; Mogenson et al. 1993; Price 1999). Such interactions are evidenced by findings that defensive behaviors and cardiovascular responses evoked by electrical stimulation of the amygdala are attenuated or abated by concomitant stimulation of orbital cortex sites, which when stimulated alone produce no autonomic changes (Timms 1977). In depressed humans, orbital metabolism correlates inversely with amygdala metabolism, possibly also reflecting the modulatory influence of orbital activity on amygdala function (Drevets 2000).

Although tumors and cerebrovascular lesions involving the frontal lobe increase the risk for developing MDE, the specific PFC regions where dysfunction confers this risk remain unclear (Mayeux 1982; Starkstein and Robinson 1989). Humans with lesions of the orbital cortex show impaired performance on tasks requiring application of information related to reward or punishment, exhibit difficulty shifting intellectual strategies in response to changing demands, and perseverate in strategies that become inappropriate (Bechara et al. 1998; Rolls 1995). Likewise, monkeys with experimental lesions of the lateral orbital cortex/VLPFC demonstrate difficulty in learning to withhold prepotent responses to nonrewarding stimuli as reinforcement contingencies change (Iversen and Mishkin 1970).

Activation of the orbital cortex during MDE may reflect endogenous attempts to attenuate emotional expression or to interrupt perseverative patterns of aversive thought and emotion. Nevertheless, evidence that neuropathological changes exist in the orbital cortex in primary mood disorders raises the possibility that these attempts are ineffective. Postmortem studies report abnormal reductions of gray matter, glia, and neuronal size in areas of the orbital cortex in MDD (Bowen et al. 1989; Rajkowska et al. 1997, 1999). If such abnormalities are associated with disturbed synaptic interactions between the orbital cortex and the amygdala, ventromedial striatum, hypothalamus, or PAG, then orbital dysfunction may contribute to the development of excessive emotional responses to stressors or ruminative ideation.

The abnormalities of serotonergic and catecholaminergic neurotransmitter function reported in mood disorders suggest other mechanisms by which orbital activity may be impaired in primary mood disorders. In healthy subjects, 5-HT depletion (via tryptophan-free diet) produced performance deficits on decision-making tasks involving risk/reward probabilities that were similar to those seen in subjects with orbital cortex lesions (Rogers et al. 1999). In addition, the depressive relapse occurring in remitted MDD subjects scanned during serotonin depletion was associated with reductions in metabolism in the orbital cortex and VLPFC (Bremner et al. 1997; the area termed "middle frontal" by Bremner is part of the VLPFC area described herein). Finally, the orbital cortex metabolism is decreased in depressed versus nondepressed subjects with Parkinson's disease, suggesting that dopamine depletion may also impair orbital cortex function (Mayberg et al. 1990; Ring et al. 1994).

The effects of antidepressant treatment on neurophysiological activity in the orbital cortex and VLPFC are noteworthy in this regard. The highly replicated finding that CBF and metabolism decrease in the orbital/insular cortex and VLPFC during effective antidepressant treatment may indicate that this cortex can "relax" because such treatments directly inhibit pathological limbic activity (reviewed in Drevets 1999). In contrast, nonpharmacological antidepressant treatments such as cognitive behavioral therapy and rTMS reportedly *increase* metabolism in the VLPFC/anterior insula and posterior orbital cortex, respectively (Brody et al. 2001; Teneback et al. 1999), suggesting the hypothesis that their therapeutic mechanisms depend on enhancing the function of PFC mechanisms for attenuating emotional expression.

Dorsomedial/Dorsal Anterolateral Prefrontal Cortex

Other PFC regions where dysfunction may impair the ability to modulate emotional responses in mood disorders include the dorsomedial PFC (DMPFC; vicinity of dorsal Brodmann area [BA] 32 and rostral BA 9) and dorsal anterolateral PFC (DALPFC; approximately rostral BA 9). Several PET studies of MDD found abnormally decreased resting CBF and metabolism in these areas, which normalized during effective antidepressant therapy in some but not other studies (Baxter et al. 1989; Drevets et al. 1999b). Ring et al. (1994) showed that CBF is also reduced in the DMPFC in depressed versus nondepressed subjects with Parkinson's disease. In postmortem studies of MDD, Rajkowska et al. (1999) observed abnormal reductions in the density and size of neurons and glia in the supra- and infragranular layers of rostral 9, a finding that may relate to the reduction in metabolic activity in this area in PET studies of depression.

In brain mapping studies of healthy humans, CBF in the DMPFC increases as subjects perform tasks that elicit emotional responses or require emotional evaluations (Dolan et al. 1996; Drevets et al. 1994; Reiman et al. 1997). In healthy humans imaged during anticipation of an electrical shock, the relationship between CBF and emotion ratings suggested that although this region activated during anxiety, it exerted a modulatory influence on emotional expression, such that the change in anxiety ratings and heart rate correlated inversely with CBF (Drevets et al. 1994). In rats, lesions of the area that appears homologous with the human DMPFC result in exaggerated heart rate responses to fear-conditioned stimuli, and electrical and chemical stimulation of these sites attenuates defensive behavior and cardiovascular responses evoked by amygdala stimulation (reviewed in Frysztak and Neafsey 1994). The DMPFC sends efferent projections to the PAG, through which it may modulate cardiovascular responses associated with emotional behavior or stress (Price 1999). If the histopathological changes found in this area in MDD by Rajkowska et al. (1999) are associated with functional impairment, then they may conceivably contribute to development of pathological emotional behavior in MDD.

Dorsolateral Prefrontal/Dorsal Anterior Cingulate Cortex

Abnormal reductions of CBF and metabolism have also been reported in MDD in areas of the lateral and DLPFC and dorsal anterior cingulate cortex situated posterior to the areas described in the preceding section (reviewed in Drevets and Raichle 1998; Drevets et al. 1999b). These abnormalities appear mood-state–dependent, and reverse during symptom remission (Baxter et al. 1989; Bench et al. 1995; Mayberg et al. 1999). Initial MRI and neuropathological studies have not identified abnormalities of cortex volume or cell counts in these regions in primary mood disorders (Bowen et al. 1989; Drevets et al. 1997; Rajkowska et al. 1997).

Human PET and fMRI studies show that hemodynamic responses in the anterior cingulate cortex dorsal and posterior to the genu of the corpus callosum consistently increase during tasks requiring discriminative attention and selection for action (reviewed in Drevets and Raichle 1998). Attentional demand, target frequency, and/or frequency of being incited to action modulate the magnitude of CBF in this region (reviewed in Drevets and Raichle 1998). In contrast, CBF *decreased* in this area during experimentally induced anxiety in healthy subjects (Drevets and Raichle 1998). As described earlier, this phenomenon may reflect cross-modal suppression of neural transmission related to unattended cognitive or behavioral processes. Consistent with the possibility that this phenomenon reflects a competitive interaction between cognitive and emotional processing (Drevets and Raichle 1998), Dolan et al. (1994) showed that the reduction in CBF in this region correlates with cognitive impairment in depressed subjects.

Brain mapping studies indicate that areas of the lateral and dorsolateral PFC activate when verbal or visuospatial information is maintained in working memory and processed in some way (Buckner and Tulving 1995; Goldman-Rakic 1987). In the vicinity of these areas, CBF and metabolism are reportedly decreased in the depressed to the remitted phase of MDD, in depressed subjects relative to healthy control subjects, and during experimentally induced sadness in healthy subjects (Bench et al. 1992; Biver et al. 1994; Mayberg et al. 1999). These DLPFC areas do not appear activated during emotional processing, and lesions of this region do not impair performance on tasks involving the application of information related to rewarding or aversive stimuli (e.g., Bechara et al. 1998). Dolan et al. (1993) reported that the reduction in CBF in the DLPFC instead correlates with impoverishment of speech in both MDD and schizophrenia and may thus reflect slowing of cognitive processes involving these regions.

Abnormalities in Striatum, Thalamus, and Other Brain Areas

The amygdala and the orbital, ventrolateral, and subgenual PFC share extensive anatomical connections with the mediodorsal nucleus of the thalamus (MNT) and the ventromedial striatum (Nauta and Domesick 1984; Price 1999; Price et al. 1996). In the left medial thalamus, CBF and metabolism are abnormally increased in depressed subjects with MDD or BD (Figure 6-4; Drevets et al. 1992, 1995b). In contrast, CBF and metabolism are abnormally decreased in the caudate in MDD (Baxter et al. 1985; Drevets et al. 1992). The volume of the caudate head and ventral striatum appear abnormally decreased in MRI and postmortem studies of MDD (Baumann et al. 1999; Krishnan et al. 1992). Partial volume effects of this morphometric reduction in caudate size may thus account for the CBF and metabolic reductions in this area in MDD.

Regional CBF and metabolic abnormalities in other structures have been less consistently replicated. Abnormally increased CBF has been reported in the posterior cingulate cortex and medial cerebellum in MDD (Bench et al. 1992; Buchsbaum et al. 1997). Medial cerebellar CBF also increases during experimentally induced anxiety or sadness in healthy or anxiety-disordered subjects (reviewed in Drevets and Botteron 1997; George et al.

1995). Some studies report reduced CBF and metabolism in lateral temporal and inferior parietal areas implicated in sensory processing in MDD (e.g., Biver et al. 1994; Cohen et al. 1992; Drevets et al. 1992). Deactivation of such areas during depressive episodes may reflect phenomena similar to those discussed earlier for the lateral/dorsolateral PFC and may relate to neuropsychological deficits in MDD (Drevets and Raichle 1998).

ANATOMICAL CIRCUITS IMPLICATED IN MDD

The abnormalities of structure and function in mood disorders implicate limbic-thalamo-cortical (LTC) circuits, involving the amygdala, medial thalamus, and orbital and medial PFC, as well as limbic-cortical-striatal-pallidal-thalamic (LCSPT) circuits, involving the components of the LTC circuit along with related parts of the striatum and pallidum (Figure 6-5; Drevets et al. 1992). The amygdala and PFC are interconnected by excitatory projections with each other and with the MNT (Carmichael and Price 1995; Price et al. 1996). Through these connections, the amygdala is in a position to directly activate the PFC and to modulate the reciprocal interaction between the PFC and MNT (e.g., Garcia et al. 1999), potentially accounting for the increased metabolic activity in the LTC during MDE (Drevets et al. 1992).

Pathologically increased amygdala activity could also produce abnormal activity in the PFC and MNT through the striatum and pallidum. The amygdala and PFC send excitatory projections to overlapping parts of the ventromedial caudate and nucleus accumbens (Carmichael and Price 1995; Nauta and Domesick 1984; Price et al. 1996). This part of the striatum sends inhibitory projections to the ventral pallidum, which in turn sends GABA-ergic, inhibitory fibers to the MNT (Graybiel 1990). Because the pallidal neurons have relatively high spontaneous firing rates (De Long 1972), activity in the amygdala or PFC that activates the striatum and in turn inhibits the ventral pallidum may release the MNT from an inhibitory pallidal influence.

As described above, the putative role of the orbital and medial PFC in modulating emotional and stress responses could potentially be disturbed either at the level of the PFC or at the level of these PFC regions' efferent projection fields in the striatum. Consistent with this hypothesis, both lesions of the PFC and of the striatum (e.g., strokes or tumors) and degenerative diseases involving the striatum (e.g., Parkinson's and Huntington's diseases) are associated with higher rates of secondary major depression than similarly debilitating conditions that spare these regions (Folstein et al. 1991; Mayeux 1982; Starkstein and Robinson 1989). Because these conditions affect the LCSPT and LTC circuitry in different ways, imbalances within these circuits, rather than overall increased or decreased synaptic activity in a particular structure, may increase the risk for developing MDE (Drevets et al. 1992).

Implications of Neuropathological Findings in LTC and LCSPT Circuits

In primary MDD and BD, histopathological changes have been identified in multiple parts of the LTC and LCSPT circuits that may disturb their modulatory influence over emotional behavior (Figure 6-5).

Postmortem assessments of the subgenual PFC (agranular cortex on the prelimbic portion of the anterior cingulate gyrus [part of BA 24]) and posterior orbital cortex demonstrated an abnormal reduction in gray matter (consistent with the in vivo MRI findings of Drevets et al. [1997]) that was associated with a *reduction* in glia and no equivalent loss of neurons in MDD and BD relative to healthy and schizophrenic control samples (Öngür et al. 1998; Rajkowska et al. 1999). In addition, Bowley et al. (2000) recently reported that the glial cell number and density and the glia-to-neuron ratio were abnormally decreased in the amygdala in MDD subjects studied postmortem. In the ventral striatum, postmortem assessments showed decreased volume in MDD and BD samples relative to control subjects, although the histopathological correlates of this abnormality were not reported (Baumann et al. 1999). Finally, the thalamic and hypothalamic areas that receive projections from the orbital and medial PFC may also be affected because the third ventricle is enlarged in adults and adolescents with BD (reviewed in Drevets and Botteron 1997). In contrast, the volume of the whole brain, the entire PFC, the dorsal anterior cingulate, the somatosensory cortex, the lateral temporal cortex, and other control regions have not differed between midlife- or early-onset MDD or BD subjects and healthy control subjects (e.g., Drevets et al. 1997; Pearlson et al. 1997). Morphometric data in the hippocampus have been less clear, as subtle reductions of hippocampal volume were found by some but not most MRI studies of MDD or BD, and histopathological assessments of the hippocampus have thus far been negative (reviewed in Drevets et al. 1999a, 1999b).

Although the etiology and time course of these abnormalities are unknown, the histopathology and the apparent specificity for areas implicated in the modulation of emotional behavior suggest clues regarding their pathogenesis. The histopathological changes imply these volumetric deficits are accounted for by reductions in neuropil rather than by neurodegenerative processes. Glia are dividing cells that support neurons and synaptic transmission, so the reduction in glia may conceivably arise secondary to a loss or underdevelopment of synapses (Magistretti et al. 1995). Nevertheless, because glia transport glutamate and GABA from the extracellular fluid and provide trophic factors and energy substrates to neurons, glial hypofunction may also disturb synaptic transmission within the affected cortex and contribute to a reduction in neuropil (Azmitia 1999; Magistretti et al. 1995).

The neuropil volume reflects the number of neuritic processes that can be modulated in some regions of the adult brain by exposure to increased concentrations of excitatory amino acid neurotransmitters or cortisol and by decreased function of factors that maintain the cytoskeleton such as neurotrophin expression, and serotonin 1A (5-HT_{1A}) and estrogen receptor stimulation (Azmitia 1999; Coyle and Puttfarcken 1993; Duman et al. 1997; McEwen 1999). For example, chronic exposure to relatively small elevations in excitatory amino acid neurotransmitter (i.e., glutamate) or cortisol concentrations can induce "dendritic reshaping" in which dendrites retract, presumably reducing neuropil volume (McEwen 1999). This process has been best characterized in the hippocampus; however, the extent to which it occurs in the cerebral cortex, basal ganglia, and other limbic structures remains unclear.

In primary mood disorders, abnormally elevated cortisol concentrations and reduced 5-HT_{1A} receptor function may be risk factors for developing reductions in neuropil that could affect widespread regions (e.g., Drevets et al. 1999a; Lopez et al. 1998; Musselman and Nemeroff 1993; Sargent et al. 2000; Young et al. 1993). However, the targeted nature of the gray matter volume reductions to specific areas of the LTC and LCSPT circuits (e.g., left, but not right, subgenual PFC; Drevets et al. 1997; Hirayasu et al. 1999; Figure 6-5) suggests that glutamatergic neurotransmission may play a major role in inducing neuropil alterations in primary mood disorders. The finding that during MDE, regional CBF and metabolism are elevated in the LTC pathway, which is formed by predominantly glutamatergic projections, suggests a potential source for chronic glutamate exposure (Drevets et al. 1992). Glutamate is predominantly removed from the extracellular fluid by transporter sites situated on the astroglial endfeet, which encompass synapses (Magistretti et al. 1995). However, if the reduction of astroglia found in mood disorders (Rajkowska et al. 2000) impairs the efficiency of glutamate transport, it is conceivable that glutamate concentrations may increase. The potential excitotoxic effects of elevated glutamate concentrations may be facilitated in affective illness by increased release of cortisol, which antagonizes glutamate transport (Sapolsky 1996; Young et al. 1993).

Currently, the only evidence that glutamate transport may be insufficient in depression is that high-affinity NMDA glutamatergic receptors are downregulated in the PFC of suicide victims, compatible with antemortem exposure to excessive glutamate concentrations (Nowak et al. 1995). It is nevertheless noteworthy that antidepressant treatments may compensate for impaired glutamate transport, as repeated electroconvulsive shock and chronic antidepressant administration desensitize NMDA-glutamatergic receptors in the rat frontal cortex (Paul et al. 1994), and some anticonvulsant agents that are effective in BD reduce glutamatergic transmission (Sporn and Sachs 1997). The more recently discovered neurotrophic and neuroprotective effects of chronic antidepressant and mood-stabilizing treatments may also play roles in ameliorating the neuromorphometric changes in primary mood disorders (Duman et al. 1997; Manji et al. 1999).

Finally, the reported antidepressant drug effects of increasing serotonin transmission, tonically activating postsynaptic 5-HT$_{1A}$ receptors, and enhancing negative feedback inhibition of cortisol release may protect against or reverse neuropil reduction (Chaput et al. 1991; Duman et al. 1997; Haddjeri et al. 1998; McEwen et al. 1999). For example, stimulation of neuron-based 5-HT$_{1A}$ receptors inhibits disassociation of the proteins that make up the long tubulin polymers that form the dendritic cytoskeleton, and stimulation of astroglial-based 5-HT$_{1A}$ receptors induces release of the neurotrophic factor S100, which promotes tubulin polymerization and inhibits breakdown of microtubules (Azmitia 1999). Conversely, administration of agents that deplete serotonin, 5-HT$_{1A}$ receptor antagonists, or antibodies to S100 all produce similar losses of dendrites, spines, and/or synapses in adult and developing animals, effects that are blocked by administration of 5-HT$_{1A}$ receptor agonists or SSRIs (Azmitia 1999).

CONCLUSION

Neuroimaging studies of primary mood disorders have identified neurophysiological abnormalities in the orbital and medial PFC, the amygdala, and related parts of the striatum and thalamus. Some of these abnormalities appear mood state dependent and are located in regions where CBF increases during normal and other pathological emotional states. These differences between depressed and control subjects may thus implicate areas where physiological activity changes to mediate or respond to the emotional, behavioral, and cognitive manifestations of MDE. Other abnormalities persist following symptom remission and are found in areas where postmortem studies demonstrate reductions in cortex volume and histopathological changes in primary mood disorders. These areas appear to modulate emotional behavior and stress responses, based on evidence from brain mapping, lesion analysis, and electrophysiological studies of humans and experimental animals. Dysfunction involving these regions is thus hypothesized to play a role in the pathogenesis of depressive symptoms. Together, these findings implicate interconnected neural circuits in which dysfunction may result in the emotional, motivational, cognitive, and behavioral manifestations of mood disorders.

REFERENCES

Abercrombie HC, Larson CL, Ward RT, et al: Metabolic rate in the amygdala predicts negative affect and depression severity in depressed patients: an FDG-PET study. Neuroimage 3:S217, 1996

Awad IA, Johnson PC, Spetzler RJ, et al: Incidental subcortical lesions identified on magnetic resonance imaging in the elderly, II: postmortem pathological correlations. Stroke 17:1090–1097, 1986

Azmitia EC: Serotonin neurons, neuroplasticity, and homeostasis of neural tissue. Neuropsyopharmacology 21(2 suppl):33S–45S, 1999

Baumann B, Danos P, Krell D, et al: Reduced volume of limbic system–affiliated basal ganglia in mood disorders: preliminary data from a postmortem study. J Neuropsychiatry Clin Neurosci 11(1):71–78, 1999

Baxter LR, Phelps ME, Mazziotta JC, et al: Cerebral metabolic rates for glucose in mood disorders. Arch Gen Psychiatry 42:441–447, 1985

Baxter LR, Phelps ME, Mazziotta JC, et al: Local cerebral glucose metabolic rates in obsessive-compulsive disorder: a comparison with rates in unipolar depression and in normal control subjects. Arch Gen Psychiatry, 44:211–218, 1987

Baxter LR, Schwartz JM, Phelps ME, et al: Reduction of prefrontal cortex glucose metabolism common to three types of depression. Arch Gen Psychiatry 46:243–250, 1989

Bechara A, Damasio H, Tranel D, et al: Dissociation of working memory from decision-making within the human prefrontal cortex. J Neurosci 18(1):428–437, 1998

Bench CJ, Friston KJ, Brown RG, et al: The anatomy of melancholia focal abnormalities of cerebral blood flow in major depression. Psychol Med 22:607–615, 1992

Bench CJ, Frackowiak RSJ, Dolan RJ: Changes in regional cerebral blood flow on recovery from depression. Psychol Med 25:247–251, 1995

Biver F, Goldman S, Delvenne V, et al: Frontal and parietal metabolic disturbances in unipolar depression. Biol Psychiatry 36:381–388, 1994

Botteron KN, Raichle ME, Heath AC, et al: An epidemiological twin study of prefrontal neuromorphometry in early-onset depression. Biol Psychiatry 45:59S, 1999

Botteron KN, Raichle ME, Drevets WC, et al: Volumetric reduction in left subgenual prefrontal cortex in early onset depression. Biol Psychiatry, in press

Bowen DM, Najlerahim A, Procter AW, et al: Circumscribed changes of the cerebral cortex in neuropsychiatric disorders of later life. Proc Natl Acad Sci U S A 86:9504–9508, 1989

Bowley MP, Drevets WC, Öngür D, et al: Glial changes in the amygdala and entorhinal cortex in mood disorders. Soc Neurosci Abstr 26:867.10, 2000

Bremner JD, Innis RB, Salomon RM, et al: Positron emission tomography measurement of cerebral metabolic correlates of tryptophan depletion–induced depressive relapse. Arch Gen Psychiatry 54:346–374, 1997

Brody AL, Saxena S, Silverman DHS, et al: Brain metabolic changes in major depressive disorder from pre- to post-treatment with paroxetine. Psychiatry Research—Neuroimaging 91:127–139, 1999a

Brody AL, Saxena S, Stoessel P, et al: Regional brain metabolic changes in patients with major depressive disorder treated with either paroxetine or interpersonal therapy. Arch Gen Psychiatry 58:631–640, 2001

Brothers L: Neurophysiology of the perception of intentions by primates, in The Cognitive Neurosciences. Edited by Gazzaniga MS. Cambridge, MA, MIT Press, 1995, pp 1107–1116

Buchsbaum MS, Wu J, Siegel BV, et al: Effect of sertraline on regional metabolic rate in patients with affective disorder. Biol Psychiatry 41:15–22, 1997

Buckner RL, Tulving E: Neuroimaging studies of memory: theory and recent PET results, in Handbook of Neuropsychology. Edited by Boller F, Grafman J. Amsterdam, The Netherlands, Elsevier, 1995, pp 439–466

Carmichael ST, Price JL: Limbic connections of the orbital and medial prefrontal cortex in Macaque monkeys. J Comp Neurol 363:615–641, 1995

Carney RM, Rich MW, teVelde A, et al: The relationship between heart rate, heart rate variability and depression in patients with coronary artery disease. J Psychosom Res 32(2):159–164, 1988

Chapin JK, Woodward DJ: Somatic sensory transmission to the cortex during movement: phasic modulation over the locomotor step cycle. Exp Neurol 78:670–684, 1982

Chapman CE, Ageranioti-Bélanger SA: Discharge properties of neurones in the hand area of primary somatosensory cortex in monkeys in relation to the performance of an active touch tactile discrimination task I: areas 3b and 1. Exp Brain Res 87:319–339, 1991

Chaput Y, deMontigny C, Blier P: Presynaptic and postsynaptic modifications of the serotonin system by long-term administration of antidepressant treatments: an in vivo electrophysiologic study in the rat. Neuropsychopharmacology 5(4):219–229, 1991

Chimowitz MI, Estes ML, Furlan AJ, et al: Further observations on the pathology of subcortical lesions identified on magnetic resonance imaging. Arch Neurol 49:747–752, 1992

Cohen RM, Gross M, Nordahl TE, et al: Preliminary data on the metabolic brain pattern of patients with winter seasonal affective disorder. Arch Gen Psychiatry 49:545–552, 1992

Coyle JT, Puttfarcken P: Oxidative stress, glutamate, and neurodegenerative disorders. Science 262:689–695, 1993

Crino PB, Morrison JH, Hof PR: Monoaminergic innervation of cingulate cortex, in Neurobiology of Cingulate Cortex and Limbic Thalamus. Edited by Vogt BA, Gabriel M. Boston, MA, Birkhauser, 1993, pp 285–312

Damasio AR, Tranel D, Damasio H: Individuals with sociopathic behavior caused by frontal damage fail to respond autonomically to social stimuli. Behav Brain Res 41:81–94, 1990

Damasio AR, Grabowski TJ, Bechara A, et al: Neural correlates of the experience of emotions. Soc Neurosci Abstr 24:258, 1998

Davis M: The role of the amygdala in conditioned fear, in The Amygdala: Neurobiological Aspects of Emotion. Edited by Aggleton JP. New York, Wiley-Liss, 1992, pp 255–305

DeLong MR: Activity of basal ganglia neurons during movement. Brain Res 40:127–135, 1972

Derdeyn CP, Yundt KD, Videen TO, et al: Increased oxygen extraction fraction is associated with prior ischemic events in patients with carotid occlusion. Stroke 29(4):754–758, 1998

Dioro D, Viau V, Meaney MJ: The role of the medial prefrontal cortex (cingulate gyrus) in the regulation of hypothalamic-pituitary-adrenal responses to stress. J Neurosci 3(9):3839–3847, 1993

DiRocco RJ, Kageyma GH, Wong-Riley MT: The relationship between CNS metabolism and cytoarchitecture: a review of ^{14}C-deoxyglucose studies with correlation to cytochrome oxidase histochemistry. Comput Med Imaging Graph 13:81–92, 1989

Dolan RJ, Bench CJ, Liddle PF, et al: Dorsolateral prefrontal cortex dysfunction in the major psychoses: symptom or disease specificity? J Neurol Neurosurg Psychiatry 56:1290–1294, 1993

Dolan RJ, Bench CJ, Brown RG, et al: Neuropsychological dysfunction in depression: the relationship to regional cerebral BF. Psychol Med 24:849–857, 1994

Dolan RJ, Fletcher P, Morris J, et al: Neural activation during covert processing of positive emotional expressions. Neuroimage 4:194–200, 1996

Drevets WC: PET and the functional anatomy of major depression, in Emotion, Memory and Behavior: Study of Human and Nonhuman Primates. Edited by Nakajima T, Taketoshi O. Tokyo, Japan, Japan Scientific Societies Press, 1995, pp 43–62

Drevets WC: Prefrontal cortical-amygdalar metabolism in major depression, in Advancing From the Ventral Striatum to the Extended Amygdala: Implications for Neuropsychiatry and Drug Abuse. Annals of the New York Academy of Sciences. New York, New York Academy of Sciences, 1999, pp 614–637

Drevets WC: Neuroimaging studies of mood disorders. Biol Psychiatry 48:813–829, 2000

Drevets WC: Neuroimaging and neuropathological studies of depression: implications for the cognitive-emotional features of mood disorders. Curr Opin Neurobiol 11:240–249, 2001

Drevets WC, Botteron K: Neuroimaging in psychiatry, in Adult Psychiatry. Edited by Guze SB. St. Louis, MO, Mosby, 1997, pp 53–81

Drevets WC, Raichle ME: Reciprocal suppression of regional cerebral blood flow during emotional versus higher cognitive processes: implications for interactions between emotion and cognition. Cognition and Emotion 12(3):353–385, 1998

Drevets WC, Todd RD: Depression, mania and related disorders, in Adult Psychiatry. Edited by Guze SB. St. Louis, MO, Mosby, 1997, pp 99–141

Drevets WC, Videen TO, Price JL, et al: A functional anatomical study of unipolar depression. J Neurosci 12:3628–3641, 1992

Drevets WC, Videen TO, Snyder AZ, et al: Regional cerebral blood flow changes during anticipatory anxiety. Abstr Soc Neurosci 20(1):368, 1994

Drevets WC, Burton H, Simpson JR, et al: Blood flow changes in human somatosensory cortex during anticipated stimulation. Nature 373:249–252, 1995a

Drevets WC, Spitznagel E, Raichle ME: Functional anatomical differences between major depressive subtypes. J Cereb Blood Flow Metab 15(1):S93, 1995c

Drevets WC, Simpson JR, Raichle ME: Regional blood flow changes in response to phobic anxiety and habituation. J Cereb Blood Flow Metab 15(1):S856, 1995b

Drevets WC, Price JL, Simpson JR, et al: Subgenual prefrontal cortex abnormalities in mood disorders. Nature 386:824–827, 1997

Drevets WC, Gadde K, Krishnan R: Neuroimaging studies of depression, in Neurobiology of Mental Illness. Edited by Charney DS, Nestler EJ, Bunney BJ. New York, Oxford University Press, 1999a, pp 394–418

Drevets WC, Frank E, Price JC, et al: PET imaging of serotonin 1A receptor binding in depression. Biol Psychiatry 46(10):1375–1387, 1999b

Duman RS, Heninger GR, Nestler EJ: A molecular and cellular theory of depression. Arch Gen Psychiatry 54:597–606, 1997

Ebert D, Feistel H, Barocka A: Effects of sleep deprivation on the limbic system and the frontal lobes in affective disorders: a study with Tc-99m-HMPAO SPECT. Psychiatry Research—Neuroimaging 40:247–251, 1991

Fazekas F: Magnetic resonance signal abnormalities in asymptomatic individuals: their incidence and functional correlates. Eur Neurol 29:164–168, 1989

Feldman S, Conforti N, Itzik A, Weidenfeld J: Differential effects of amygdaloid lesions on CRF-41, ACTH and corticosterone responses following neural stimuli. Brain Res 658:21–26, 1994

Fibiger HC: The dopamine hypotheses of schizophrenia and mood disorders, in The Mesolimbic Dopamine System: From Motivation to Action. Edited by Willner P, Scheel-Kruger J. New York, Wiley, 1991, pp 615–638

Folstein SE, Peyser CE, Starkstein SE, et al: Subcortical triad of Huntington's disease: a model for a neuropathology of depression, dementia, and dyskinesia, in Psychopathology and the Brain. Edited by Carroll BJ, Barrett. New York, Raven, 1991, pp 65–75

Francis PT, Poynton A, Lowe SL, et al: Brain amino acid concentrations and Ca^{2+}-dependent release in intractable depression assessed antemortem. Brain Res 494:314–324, 1989

Friston KJ, Frith CD, Liddle PF, et al: Comparing functional (PET) images: the assessment of significant change. J Cereb Blood Flow Metab 11:690–699, 1991

Frysztak RJ, Neafsey EJ: The effect of medial frontal cortex lesions on cardiovascular conditioned emotional responses in the rat. Brain Res 643:181–193, 1994

Garcia R, Vouimba R-M, Baudry M, et al: The amygdala modulates prefrontal cortex activity relative to conditioned fear. Nature 402:294–296, 1999

George MS, Ketter TA, Parekh PI, et al: Brain activity during transient sadness and happiness in healthy women. Am J Psychiatry 152:341–351, 1995

Gloor P, Olivier A, Quesney LF, et al: The role of the limbic system in experiential phenomena of temporal lobe epilepsy. Ann Neurol 12:129–144, 1982

Goldman-Rakic PS: Circuitry of primate prefrontal cortex and regulation of behavior by representational memory, in Handbook of Physiology: The Nervous System, Sec 1, Vol 5. Edited by Mills J, Mountcastle VB. Baltimore, MD, Williams & Wilkins, 1987, pp 373–417

Graybiel AM: Neurotransmitters and neuromodulators in the basal ganglia. Trends Neurosci 13:244–254, 1990

Haddjeri N, Blier P, de Montigny C: Long-term antidepressant treatments result in tonic activation of forebrain 5-HT1A receptors. J Neurosci 18(23):10150–10156, 1998

Haxby JV, Horwitz B, Ungerleider LG, et al: The functional organization of human extrastriate cortex: a PET-rCBF study of selective attention to faces and locations. J Neurosci 14:6336–6353, 1994

Herman JP, Cullinan WE: Neurocircuitry of stress: central control of the hypothalamo-pituitary-adrenocortical axis. Trends Neurosci 20(2):78–84, 1997

Hirayasu Y, Shenton ME, Salisbury DF, et al: Subgenual cingulate cortex volume in first-episode psychosis. Am J Psychiatry 156(7):1091–1093, 1999

Holsboer F: Neuroendocrinology of mood disorders, in Psychopharmacology: The Fourth Generation of Progress. Edited by Bloom FE, Kupfer DJ. New York, Raven, 1995, pp 957–969

Iverson SD, Mishkin M: Perseverative interference in monkeys following selective lesions of the inferior prefrontal convexity. Exp Brain Res 11:376–386, 1970

Kegeles LS, Malone KM, Slifstein M, et al: Response of cortical metabolic deficits to serotonergic challenges in mood disorders. Biol Psychiatry 45:76S, 1999

Ketter T, Kimbrell TA, Little JT, et al: Differences and commonalties in cerebral function in bipolar compared to unipolar depression. Presented at the 38th Annual Meeting of American College of Neuropsychopharmacology, Acapulco, Mexico, December 12–16, 1999

Krishnan KRR, McDonald WM, Escalona PR, et al: Magnetic resonance imaging of the caudate nuclei in depression: preliminary observations, Arch Gen Psychiatry 49:553–557, 1992

Krishnan KRR, McDonald WM, Doraiswamy PM, et al: Neuroanatomical substrates of depression in the elderly. Eur Arch Psychiatry Neurosci 243:41–46, 1993

Kupfer DJ, Targ E, Stack JL: Electroencephalographic sleep in unipolar depressive subtypes. Support for a biological and familial classification. J Nerv Ment Dis 170(8):494–498, 1992

LeDoux JE, Thompson ME, Iadecola C, et al: Local cerebral blood flow increases during auditory and emotional processing in the conscious rat. Science 221:576–578, 1983

Leichnetz GR, Astruc J: The efferent projections of the medial prefrontal cortex in the squirrel monkey (saimiri sciureus). Brain Res 109:455–472, 1976

Lewis DA, McChesney C: Tritiated imipramine binding distinguishes among subtypes of depression. Arch Gen Psychiatry 42:485–488, 1985

Links JM, Zubieta JK, Meltzer CC, et al: Influence of spatially heterogenous background activity on "hot object" quantitation in brain emission computed tomography. J Comput Assist Tomogr 20(4):680–687, 1996

López JF, Chalmers DT, Little KY, et al: Regulation of serotonin$_{1A}$, glucocorticoid, and mineralocorticoid receptor in rat and human hippocampus: implications for the neurobiology of depression. Biol Psychiatry 43:547–573, 1998

Magistretti PJ, Pellerin L, Martin JL: Brain energy metabolism: an integrated cellular perspective, in Psychopharmacology: The Fourth Generation of Progress. Edited by Bloom FE, Kupfer DJ. New York, Raven, 1995, pp 921–932

Manji HK, Moore GJ, Chen G: Lithium at 50: Have the neuroprotective effects of this unique cation been overlooked? Biol Psychiatry 46:929–940, 1999

Mayberg HS, Starkstein SE, Sadzot B, et al: Selective hypometabolism in the inferior frontal lobe in depressed patients with Parkinson's disease. Ann Neurol 28:57–64, 1990

Mayberg HS, Lewis PJ, Reginald W, et al: Paralimbic hypoperfusion in unipolar depression. J Nucl Med 35:929–934, 1994

Mayberg HS, Brannan SK, Mahurin RK, et al: Cingulate function in depression: a potential predictor of treatment response. Neuroreport 8(4):1057–1061, 1997

Mayberg HS, Liotti M, Brannan SK, et al: Reciprocal limbic-cortical function and negative mood: converging PET findings in depression and normal sadness. Am J Psychiatry 156:675–682, 1999

Mayeux R: Depression and dementia in Parkinson's disease, in Movement Disorders. Edited by Marsden CO, Fahn S. London, Butterworth, 1982, pp 75–95

McEwen BS: Stress and hippocampal plasticity. Ann Rev Neurosci 22:105–122, 1999

Mogenson GJ, Brudzynski SM, Wu M, et al: From motivation to action: a review of dopaminergic regulation of limbic → nucleus → accumbens → ventral pallidum → pedunculopontine nucleus circuitries involved in limbic-motor integration, in Limbic Motor Circuits and Neuropsychiatry. Edited by Kalivas PW, Barnes CD. London, CRC Press, 1993, pp 193–236

Morgan MA, LeDoux JE: Differential contribution of dorsal and ventral medial prefrontal cortex to the acquisition and extinction of conditioned fear in rats. Behav Neurosci 109:681–688, 1995

Murase S, Grenhoff J, Chouvet G, et al: Prefrontal cortex regulates burst firing and transmitter release in rat mesolimbic dopamine neurons. Neurosci Lett 157:53–56, 1993

Musselman DL, Nemeroff CB: The role of corticotropin-releasing factor in the pathophysiology of psychiatric disorders. Psychiatr Ann 23:676–681, 1993

Nauta WJH, Domesick V: Afferent and efferent relationships of the basal ganglia, in Function of the Basal Ganglia. CIBA Foundation Symposium 107. London, Pitman Press, 1984, pp 3–29

Nobler MS, Sackeim HA, Prohovnik I, et al: Regional cerebral BF in mood disorders, III: treatment and clinical response. Arch Gen Psychiatry 51:884–897, 1994

Nofzinger EF, Nichols TE, Meltzer CC, et al: Changes in forebrain function from waking to REM sleep in depression: preliminary analyses of [^{18}F]FDG PET studies. Psychiatry Research—Neuroimaging 91:59–78, 1999

Nowak G, Ordway GA, Paul IA: Alterations in the N-methyl-D-aspartate (NMDA) receptor complex in the frontal cortex of suicide victims. Brain Res 675:157–164, 1995

Öngür D, Drevets WC, Price JL: Glial reduction in the subgenual prefrontal cortex in mood disorders. Proc Natl Acad Sci U S A 95:13290–13295, 1998

Paul IA, Nowak G, Layer RT, et al: Adaption of the N-methyl-D-aspartate receptor complex following chronic antidepressant treatments. J Pharmacol Exp Ther 269(1):95–102, 1994

Pearlson GD, Barta PE, Powers RE, et al: Medial and superior temporal gyral volumes and cerebral asymmetry in schizophrenia versus bipolar disorder. Biol Psychiatry 41:1–14, 1997

Philpot MP, Banaerjee S, Needham-Bennett H, et al: 99mTc-HMPAO single photon emission tomography in late life depression: a pilot study of regional cerebral blood flow at rest and during a verbal fluency test. J Affect Disord 28:233–240, 1993

Poline JB, Holmes A, Worsley K, et al: Making statistical inferences, in Human Brain Function. Edited by Frackowiak R, Friston KJ, Frith CD, et al. London, Academic Press, 1997, pp 85–106

Posner MI, Presti D: Selective attention and cognitive control. Trends Neurosci 10:12–17, 1987

Price JL: Networks within the orbital and medial prefrontal cortex. Neurocase 5:231–224, 1999

Price JL, Carmichael ST, Drevets WC: Networks related to the orbital and medial prefrontal cortex: a substrate for emotional behavior? Prog Brain Res 107:523–536, 1996

Raichle ME: Circulatory and metabolic correlates of brain function in normal humans, in Handbook of Physiology: The Nervous System, Sec 1, Vol 5. Edited by Brookhart JM, Mountcastle VB. Baltimore, MD, American Physiology Society, 1987, pp 643– 674

Rajkowska G: Postmortem studies in mood disorders indicate altered numbers of neurons and glial cells. Biol Psychiatry 48:766–777, 2000

Rajkowska G, Selemon LD, Goldman-Rakic PS: Marked glial neuropathology in prefrontal cortex distinguishes bipolar disorder from schizophrenia. Schizophr Res 24:41, 1997

Rajkowska G, Miguel-Hidalgo JJ, Wei J, et al: Morphometric evidence for neuronal and glial prefrontal cell pathology in major depression. Biol Psychiatry 45(9):1085–1098, 1999

Rauch SL, Jenike MA, Alpert NM, et al: Regional cerebral blood flow measured during symptom provocation in obsessive-compulsive disorder using oxygen 15-labeled carbon dioxide and positron emission tomography. Arch Gen Psychiatry 51:62–70, 1994

Reiman EM, Lane RD, Ahern GL, et al: Neuroanatomical correlates of externally and internally generated human emotion. Am J Psychiatry 154(7):918–925, 1997

Ring HA, Bench CJ, Trimble MR, et al: Depression in Parkinson's disease: a positron emission study. Br J Psychiatry 165:333–339, 1994

Rogers RD, Everitt BJ, Baldacchino A, et al: Dissociable deficits in the decision-making cognition of chronic amphetamine abusers, opiate abusers, patients with focal damage to prefrontal cortex, and tryptophan-deleted normal volunteers: evidence for monoaminergic mechanisms. Neuropsychopharmacology 20:322–339, 1999

Rolls ET: A theory of emotion and consciousness, and its application to understanding the neural basis of emotion, in The Cognitive Neurosciences. Edited by Gazzaniga MS. Cambridge, MA, MIT Press, 1995, pp 1091–1106

Rubin RT, Mandell AJ, Crandall PH: Corticosteroid responses to limbic stimulation in man: localization of stimulus sites. Science 153:767–768, 1966

Sapolsky RM: Stress, glucocorticoids, and damage to the nervous system: the current state of confusion. Stress 1:1–19, 1996

Sargent PA, Kjaer KH, Bench CJ, et al: Brain serotonin$_{1A}$ receptor binding measured by positron emission tomography with [^{11}C]WAY-100635. Arch Gen Psychiatry 57:174–180, 2000

Schneider F, Gur RE, Alav A, et al: Mood effects on limbic blood flow correlate with emotion self-rating: a PET study with oxygen-15 labeled water. Psychiatry Research—Neuroimaging 61:265–283, 1995

Schultz W: Dopamine neurons and their role in reward mechanisms. Curr Opin Neurobiol 7:191–197, 1997

Sesack SR, Pickel VM: Prefrontal cortical efferents in the rat synapse on unlabeled neuronal targets of catecholamine terminals in the nucleus accumbens septi and on dopamine neurons in the ventral tegmental area. J Comp Neurol 320:145–160, 1992

Shulman GL, Corbetta M, Buckner RL, et al: Common blood flow changes across visual tasks, II: decreases in cerebral cortex. J Cogn Neurosci 9(5):647–662, 1997

Sporn J, Sachs G: The anticonvulsant lamotrigine in treatment-resistant manic-depressive illness. J Clin Psychopharmacol 17(3):185–189, 1997

Starkstein SE, Robinson RG: Affective disorders and cerebral vascular disease. Br J Psychiatry 154:170–182, 1989

Sullivan RM, Gratton A: Lateralized effects of medial prefrontal cortex lesions on neuroendocrine and autonomic stress responses in rats. J Neurosci 19(7):2834–2840, 1999

Taber MT, Fibiger HC: Electrical stimulation of the medial prefrontal cortex increases dopamine release in the striatum. Neuropsychopharmacology 9:271–275, 1993

Teneback CC, Nahas Z, Speer AM, et al: Changes in prefrontal cortex and paralimbic activity in depression following two weeks of daily left prefrontal TMS. J Neuropsychiatry Clin Neurosci 11:426–435, 1999

Timms RJ: Cortical inhibition and facilitation of the defense reaction. Journal of Physiology, London 266:98–99, 1977

Veith RC, Lewis N, Linares OA, et al: Sympathetic nervous system activity in major depression. Arch Gen Psychiatry 51:411–422, 1994

Whang KC, Burton H, Shulman GL: Selective attention in vibrotactile tasks: detecting the presence and absence of amplitude change. Percept Psychophys 50:157–165, 1991

Winokur G: The development and validity of familial subtypes in primary unipolar depression. Pharmacopsychiatry 15:142–146, 1982

Winokur G: All roads lead to depression: clinically homogenous, etiologically heterogenous. J Affect Disord 45:97–108, 1997

Woods RP, Masotho J, Cherry SR: MRI-PET registration with automated algorithm. J Comput Assist Tomogr 17:536–546, 1993

Wooten GF, Collins RC: Metabolic effects of unilateral lesion of the substantia nigra. J Neurosci l:285–291, 1981

Wu J, Gillin C, Buchsbaum MS, et al: Effect of sleep deprivation on brain metabolism of depressed patients. Am J Psychiatry 149:538–543, 1992

Young EA, Kotun J, Haskett RF, et al: Dissociation between pituitary and adrenal suppression to dexamethasone in depression. Arch Gen Psychiatry 50:395–403, 1993

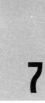

7

Genetic Neuroimaging

Helping to Define Phenotypes in Affective Disorders

Kelly N. Botteron, M.D.

It is increasingly clear that recurrent major depressive disorder (MDD) is associated with changes in brain structure and function. A growing number of studies support that there are structural and functional alterations in specific orbital and medial prefrontal limbic circuits associated with affective disorders. It is also evident that major depression and bipolar affective disorder (BAD) are not homogeneous disorders but may occur in the context of different specific etiologies. However, currently it is difficult to empirically define specific subtypes of affective disorders. Neuroimaging has the potential to assist in the phenotypic description or definition of taxonomy for disorders of interest and, as illustrated in this chapter, may have specific relevance for the phenotypic description of affective disorders. Twin or family studies serve as a useful research strategy for the clarification of etiologic heterogeneity. Furthermore, twin or family genetic designs can help to refine the definition of structural and functional brain differences and determine the nature of the changes, including differentiating the contribution of genetic or environmental factors to the alterations associated with mood disorders.

This work was supported by National Institute of Mental Health Grant MH 01292 and the National Alliance for Research on Schizophrenia and Affective Disorders.

This chapter reviews the evidence that suggests specific medial and or-bital prefrontal subcortical limbic structures are involved in the pathophys-iology of affective disorders and may be important in defining phenotypic heterogeneity. Advantages for the combined use of twin or family studies and neuroimaging are outlined. Strategies are discussed using family or twin designs to determine whether 1) changes are present prior to the onset of disorder-representing neurodevelopmental changes, 2) the onset of dis-order alters normal neurodevelopmental patterns, or 3) neurodegenerative changes occur after the onset of disorder. Finally, strategies for examining genetic or environmental contributions to differences in brain structure or function are outlined. Information obtained concurrently from these strategies provides information critical to the delineation of etiologically homogeneous subtypes of affective disorders.

IMPORTANCE OF CLARIFYING PHENOTYPIC HETEROGENEITY

A framework for defining specific diagnosis in psychiatry was eloquently delineated by Robins and Guze (1970). This definition of diagnostic clas-sification is based on criteria rooted in the tradition of general medicine and was a radical change, revolutionizing the field of psychiatric diagno-sis. Their interest in specific criteria for the definition of diagnoses was based on their belief that manifestations of psychiatric disease represented distinct categories of illness with specific underlying etiologies. Although specific etiologies were unknown for virtually all psychiatric conditions at the time, they recognized that an organized system of diagnosis was crucial to empirically study psychiatric disorders. Robins and Guze out-lined how the validity of any diagnostic categorization needed to be based on the following five criteria: 1) a consistent pattern of clinical signs and symptoms, 2) typical longitudinal clinical course over time, 3) evidence of familiality, 4) characteristic response to treatment, and 5) associated ab-normalities in laboratory or diagnostic tests. This definition has resulted in increased clarity and replicability in research, and continues to be the benchmark for psychiatric diagnostic definitions. Associated laboratory features have remained elusive for most disorders because there have been few tools available to specifically examine neuropathology associated with psychiatric disorders.

There is substantial genetic influence on the development of mood dis-orders. This is supported by a large number of family, sibling, and twin studies. Along with the recognition of this increased genetic risk, it is seen as increasingly important to identify genes related to the risk for, and expression of, major depression and BAD. The identification of specific

genes associated with risk for the expression of mood disorders will provide for more relevant descriptions of pathophysiology and could provide
important data for the development of new, genetically specific interventions, such as medications to ameliorate enzymatic insufficiencies or
drugs that are more specific to receptor subtypes. Although numerous
linkage studies have been reported, replication has been inconsistent. A
few findings have been replicated, including linkage with serotonin receptor polymorphisms and seasonal affective disorder (SAD). However, it
is increasingly clear that etiologic heterogeneity exists in individuals diagnosed with MDD. As is the case in some other disorders, a number of
specific genetic mutations might be identified as representing relatively
distinct etiologies that may converge into common physiologic pathways.
It is increasingly clear that the factors hindering the identification of genes
related to psychiatric disorders are not related to molecular genetic technology but to phenotypic description of disorders in order to accurately
characterize taxonomy (Rice and Todorov 1994; Tsuang et al. 1993). Rice
(1993) noted that etiologic heterogeneity, related to the possibility of multiple pathways leading to indistinguishable symptoms and clinical disorder,
was a major factor in the difficulty that researchers had in establishing and
replicating genetic linkage for specific disorders. Etiologic heterogeneity
has been a problem for genetics in many areas of medicine and has been
greatly ameliorated in other specialties based on the use of adjunctive laboratory, imaging, or other diagnostic data. Currently, in psychiatry, we are
usually restricted to the initial stage of differential diagnosis based on clinical symptoms and family history information alone, with only limited data
available based on laboratory, electrophysiological, or imaging studies to
differentiate the likely heterogeneous conditions represented. Molecular
genetics will eventually identify some genotypically homogenous groups;
however, the very problem of clinical, phenotypic heterogeneity hinders
the identification of specific genetic linkages. Genetic imaging studies using family and twin designs should help to define diagnostic phenotype.

ADVANTAGES OF NEUROIMAGING FOR GENETIC STUDIES

Imaging studies offer several advantages as an adjunct to genetic linkage
or association studies. First, quantitative neuroimaging data may improve
the phenotypic description of specific disorders and provide a method
to further clarify diagnostic heterogeneity based on patterns of neuromorphometric differences in individuals with phenotypically similar clinical
presentations. Second, imaging studies represent a more direct way of examining or establishing the connection between the genetic influence on

the phenotypic expression of a disorder and the underlying associated pathophysiology. Even in an ideal situation, where a specific mutation may be identified for a disorder of interest, it will continue to be important to understand and characterize the pathophysiologic mechanisms of how genetic risk affects normal brain structure and function. Quantification of deviation from normal developmental patterns will also be important in the assessment and monitoring of currently available and proposed novel treatments. Third, imaging studies provide quantitative traits that can greatly increase the power of linkage analysis (Tsuang et al. 1993). Finally, definition of regional abnormalities alone or in concert with subsequent focused neuropathology or other neurobiological studies will suggest candidate genes for investigation.

Prefrontal Limbic Circuits Associated With Affective Disorders

The neural circuits underlying normal affective expression and function are now reasonably well defined. These circuit models of affective regulation are based on an impressively diverse array of animal and human studies investigating normal affective recognition and expression, as well as regions involved in affective disorders such as major depression and mania. Converging evidence from these studies, including structural and functional imaging studies and lesion studies, demonstrates that specific interconnected regions in prefrontal (orbital prefrontal, medial prefrontal), limbic (anterior cingulate and amygdala), striatal, and thalamic structures are important in affective regulation. These same regions also appear to be important in the pathophysiology of affective disorders; this is based on substantial data demonstrating abnormalities in function, structure, and chemical composition in these brain regions. A simplified circuit model is illustrated in Figure 7-1. These circuits involve substantial reciprocal interaction between subcortical and cortical regions.

Although the literature is somewhat conflicting, many positron emission tomography (PET) imaging studies in clinical populations during an episode of MDD have reported increased cerebral blood flow (CBF) and metabolism in the ventral prefrontal cortex, anterior cingulate, amygdala, and medial thalamus, whereas CBF is reduced in the subgenual medial prefrontal cortex and striatum (Drevets 1999; George et al. 1997; Mayberg et al. 1997, 1999; Sackeim et al. 1990). Early structural imaging studies also reported conflicting results; however, similar to early PET studies, they also had significant technical limitations, which may have resulted in Type II errors. Despite the conflicting results, there is support for neuromorphometric differences in MDD and bipolar disorder, including lateral and third

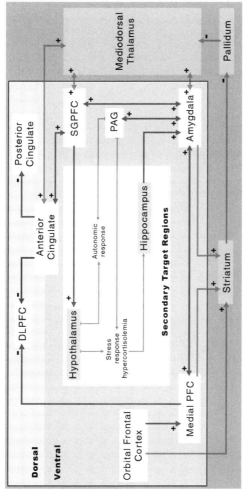

FIGURE 7-1 Simplified circuit model of regions important in affective regulation and mood disorders. Major cortical and subcortical regions are depicted. Excitatory (+) and inhibitory (−) inputs are indicated. Regions within the shaded box are primary cortical and subcortical regions involved in affective processing. Regions within the central white box are hypothesized more as secondary target regions. DLPFC = dorsolateral prefrontal cortex; SGPFC = subgenual prefrontal cortex; medial PFC = medial prefrontal cortex; PAG = periaqueductal gray matter.

ventricular enlargement and reduction in some prefrontal and temporal regions and in caudate volumes (Botteron and Figiel 1997; Soares and Mann 1997). Recent advances in magnetic resonance imaging (MRI) technology and image analysis have allowed for the more precise volumetric definition of smaller anatomical regions. Using these improved methods, a number of investigators have identified structural differences in regions in the proposed prefrontal-limbic-striatal-pallidal-thalamic circuits.

Based on the definition and understanding of these circuits (see Figure 7-1), it is evident how different specific etiologies could result in similar clinical presentations through disruption in normal homeostasis leading to affective dysregulation. Data from a variety of lesion studies, including poststroke studies, support this theory. For example, it is well established that strokes in specific regions are associated with significantly elevated rates of poststroke MDD or mania. Depression following a stroke is significantly more likely to occur if the cerebrovascular lesion is located in the left prefrontal lobe, and the incidence of secondary stroke increases as the proximity to the frontal pole increases (Robinson 1997; Robinson and Starkstein 1990; Robinson et al. 1988). Strokes in the right parietal region are also associated with an elevated but lower relative risk (Robinson 1997). In addition to the poststroke literature, it has been noted for some time that MDD occurs at significantly increased rates in a number of other specific neurologic disorders. Disorders primarily involving the basal ganglia, such as Parkinson's or Huntington's disease, are associated with substantially elevated rates of depression (Mayberg et al. 1990, 1992). A very high percentage of strokes in the basal ganglia are associated with secondary depression (Robinson 1997). The regional specificity of risk for depression secondary to other neurologic disorders also supports that disruption in specific regions in this circuit may lead to affective dysregulation, which appears phenotypically very similar to primary major depression, despite clear differences in the underlying neuropathology. We hypothesize that there may also be regionally specific patterns of functional or structural differences associated with primary mood disorders that may not be differentiated based on clinical description alone but that would be identifiable based on patterns of quantitative neuromorphometric data.

For example, it has been demonstrated in a subtype of MDD, familial pure depressive disorder, that there is reduction in volume in the left subgenual prefrontal cortex (Drevets et al. 1997). We have also demonstrated reduction in this same region in an epidemiologically identified population of young females with early-onset MDD (Botteron et al., in press), and it has also been demonstrated in adults with BAD (Hirayasu et al. 1999). Furthermore, these findings have been confirmed in neuropathology studies and were most significantly present in cases with a family history of depression (Öngür et al. 1998).

Establishing Pathophysiology Associated With Genetic Risk

The definition of specific regional brain abnormalities, alone or in concert with subsequent focused neuropathology or additional imaging studies such as spectroscopy, can help to suggest candidate genes for investigation. For example, as mentioned above, decreased subgenual prefrontal cortex volume has been demonstrated in MDD and bipolar disorder, as defined from MRI studies (Botteron et al., in press; Drevets et al. 1997; Hirayasu et al. 1999). In addition, decreased glial cell numbers are found in neuropathology studies of subjects with familial MDD or BAD in analogous regions (Öngür et al. 1998; Rajkowska et al. 1999). Some studies have suggested that neurons in this region are also somewhat smaller, although not significantly reduced in number (Rajkowska et al. 1999). Changes in glial cell number and regional volume appear to be more prominent in cases with a family history of affective disorder, suggesting that reduced glial cell number may be a genetically transmissible process. We hypothesize that similar glial cell changes would be demonstrated most consistently in cases with strongly positive family histories. An increase in familial prevalence of mood disorders has been demonstrated in early-onset depression (Neuman et al. 1997). Although currently we cannot directly measure glial cell volume, the glial changes appear to be related to decreased regional volume, which can be measured by MRI. Identification of specific regions or patterns of differences may lead to the suggestion of specific candidate genes such as glial-specific proteins, glial-associated growth factors, or regionally specific developmental factors. Glial pathology could also relate to hypotheses of serotonin dysregulation in depression because glia have substantial numbers of serotonin receptors and express serotonin transporters on their surface. Changes in serotonin receptor function associated with glia are associated with changes in glial functioning and glial development, further supporting the potential role of serotonin-related genes as important candidate genes in affective disorders.

Augmentation for Linkage Analysis Studies

The identification of specific gene mutation or specific polymorphisms associated with MDD will provide the gold standard for defining diagnostically homogeneous groups. The ability to characterize quantitative non-symptom-based parameters with disease specificity can significantly improve the power of linkage analyses. Neuroimaging parameters are ideal candidates. It is clear that there are significant limitations with phenotypic description based on clinical characteristics and family history data. It is important to recall that what we measure with the clinical description of a major depressive episode (MDE) is an imperfect indicator of the underlying pathophysiology in which we are really interested. Neuroimaging studies attempt a more direct measure of structural changes in brain regions that are known to be important in the regulation of normal affect and stress response.

Recognizing the limitations of symptomatic description alone, Tsuang et al. (1993) outlined criteria for defining additional phenotypic variables for use in genetic linkage studies. They suggested six specific guidelines for creating phenotypic identification studies for genetic studies of psychopathology: 1) specificity, 2) state independence, 3) heritability, 4) familial association, 5) cosegregation, and 6) biological plausibility. These guidelines are relevant and applicable to neuroimaging parameters for potential genetic linkage studies.

To demonstrate *specificity*, the indicator should be more strongly associated with the disease of interest in comparison to other psychiatric conditions. *State independence* is defined as a variable that is stable over time and not an epiphenomenon of the illness or its treatment. The indicator should demonstrate *heritability* and *familial association* (i.e., the indicator is more prevalent among the relatives of the ill probands than among the relatives of appropriate control subjects). *Cosegregation* is defined as the demonstration that the indicator is more prevalent among the ill relatives of the ill probands than among the well relatives of the ill probands. Finally, the proposed phenotypic variable should have *biological plausibility*, that is, the variable should have some proposed pathophysiologic relevance for the disorder of interest. As an extension related to childhood or early-onset disorders, Hudziak (1996) proposed several additional guidelines, including developmental, gender and multi-informant sensitivity.

Although a number of imaging paradigms may contribute to the understanding of disease specificity, state independence, and biological plausibility, family or twin studies of brain imaging differences are implicitly required to establish heritability, familial association, and cosegregation. Furthermore, family or twin designs offer advantages to elucidating specificity and state independence. For example, in relation to specificity, regional brain differences can be studied across disorders in standardized fashion to establish disease specificity. Evidence for specificity in the pattern of neuromorphometric differences is beginning to emerge for a number of disorders, such as affective, schizophrenic, and attentional disorders. Although bipolar disorder and schizophrenia demonstrate some common regional differences, such as increased lateral and third ventricles and changes in basal ganglia, they also demonstrate disease specificity for several regions, such as increased amygdala volume in bipolar I disorder but not schizophrenia (Altshuler et al. 2000) and decreased left superior temporal gyrus volume in schizophrenia but not bipolar I disorder (Pearlson et al. 1997). Family and twin studies provide the potential to identify more subtle regional structural imaging differences, due to reduction in variability in related individuals in comparison to general population matched control subjects.

As discussed in more detail later in this chapter, the issue of a stable indicator that is not an epiphenomenon of illness is an issue that can be most efficiently specified through the use of family and twin studies. However, in studies of childhood psychiatric disorders, there are few, if any, indicators that remain stable over time as children and adolescents display developmental changes in virtually all physical, neurological, physiological, and behavioral parameters during development. It may be more appropriate to consider looking for indicators that maintain a characteristic or abnormal developmental trajectory over time. Thus, additional guidelines proposed by Hudziak (1996), including developmental and gender specificity, are also relevant to genetic imaging studies. We hypothesize that neurodevelopmental patterns (Giedd et al. 1996; Reiss et al. 1996) will be altered in subjects with some early-onset psychiatric disorders such as affective disorders. Therefore, it is crucial to characterize neurodevelopmental patterns in regions of interest in both subjects with MDD and control subjects. This is optimally delineated with longitudinal twin or family studies (see below). Finally, gender specificity is relevant and important in most neurobiological and imaging studies and is clearly a relevant factor in MDD. That is, gender-related differences in brain structure, function, and normal neurodevelopmental patterns (Giedd et al. 1997) have been demonstrated.

ADVANTAGES OF TWIN OR FAMILY DESIGNS FOR NEUROIMAGING INVESTIGATIONS

Improved Sensitivity for Detection of Disease-Related Differences

There are several advantages associated with family or twin designs for neuroimaging investigations. The inclusion of family members with and without illness as a comparison control group can improve the sensitivity to detect subtle structural differences associated with an illness. This is so because of the significant reduction in variability of regional brain structure in genetically related individuals in comparison to matched unrelated control subjects. For example, there are a number of studies that have examined potential hippocampal volume differences associated with schizophrenia. Results from these studies have often been conflicting, with many early studies reporting no differences and mixed findings in case control studies

(McCarley et al. 1999). However, a study of monozygotic twins discordant for schizophrenia demonstrated a clear association between schizophrenia and reduced hippocampal volume when comparisons were made of affected and unaffected twins (Suddath et al. 1990). Subsequently, more sophisticated image analysis methods with higher resolution have confirmed that there is reduced hippocampal volume using traditional case control studies, and newer studies including high dimensional shape analysis have further supported the presence of structural hippocampal abnormalities in schizophrenia (Csernansky et al. 1998). However, the number of early conflicting results is a good illustration of Type II error reporting that can result when effects of small magnitude are studied in populations with high variability in the parameter of interest.

Identification of At-Risk Differences

The ideal family or twin design should include both probands with identified illness and their siblings (both affected and unaffected) and control probands without the illness of interest and their control siblings. Using this design, it is possible to identify changes associated with being at increased genetic risk of an illness, as well as structural or functional changes specifically related to illness. For example, Weinberger et al. (1981) reported that unaffected and first-degree relatives of schizophrenics have significantly larger lateral ventricles than unrelated control subjects. Other regions clearly affected in schizophrenia, such as the planum temporale or temporal lobe, have been reported to not demonstrate any differences in their unaffected relatives (Frangou et al. 1997; Honer et al. 1994; Staal et al. 2000). Studies of discordant twins can be particularly powerful in developing populations such as children or adolescents because other family members will be at different maturational stages and ongoing structural or functional development is occurring until at least young adulthood. The identification of neuropathologic or neurophysiologic abnormalities, which predate the symptomatic onset of mood disorders, would be important for early intervention, and could provide quantitative at-risk factors for the management and potential prevention or delay of onset of disorder.

Specification of Neurodevelopmental Versus Neurodegenerative Hypotheses

One significant advantage of twin or family study designs for neuroimaging investigations is the inclusion of individuals at high risk to optimally characterize neurodevelopmental versus neurodegenerative models. In major depression, there is limited evidence in support of both neuro-developmental and neurodegenerative models for structural and functional brain changes. Neurodevelopmental models were proposed in the mid-1980s and early 1990s. These models were based in part on MRI and computed tomography (CT) data, suggesting limbic structural differences that, in some cases, are similar to those reported in schizophrenia. The pattern of these changes was considered consistent with a neurodevelopmental etiology in both disorders. However, there are also data supporting that some changes associated with MDD may be related to neurodegenerative mechanisms. The best example of this is the demonstration of reduced hippocampal volume (Bremner et al. 2000; Sheline et al. 1996), which has been reported by some but not all investigators (Vakili et al. 2000). Methodological considerations may have contributed to the disparate findings.

More recent studies—with the highest resolution images, anatomically correct definition, and improved image analysis methods—have more consistently reported reduced hippocampal volume. For example, hippocampal volume reduction was correlated with estimates of the total lifetime length of depressive episodes (Bremner 1999; Sheline et al. 1996). It has been hypothesized that this reduction could be related to secondary effects of depression, including effects of excitotoxic injury related to cortisol dysregulation (Bremner 1999; Sapolsky et al. 1985, 1986). The cortisol-related, excitotoxic hypotheses are further supported by animal studies with rat and primate models of affective disorders (including learned helplessness models), demonstrating that cortisol dysregulation leads to neuronal loss and atrophy in specific brain regions, including the hippocampus. Whether hippocampal volume loss in subjects with depression is a neurodegenerative process remains an open question. There have not been any longitudinal results reported to date, and there has been little reported concerning younger subjects with depression.

It is ideal to examine twin and family study designs if regions that are potentially sensitive to the ongoing effects of illness do not differ from control subjects prior to the phenotypic onset of illness but do begin to demonstrate structural changes following the onset of MDD. Such a pattern would be consistent with a degenerative process. Alternatively, it could be hypothesized that there is preexisting vulnerability in specific regions that subsequently results in neurodegenerative changes following a second "hit" related to environmental factors or onset of illness. This hypothesis would postulate that structures such as the hippocampus would demonstrate subtle differences predating the onset of illness, and later demonstrate additional neurodegenerative changes after the onset of illness. Differentiating these models will be important in understanding the pathophysiology of depression and will have important implications for

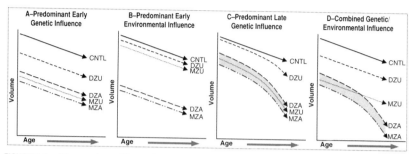

FIGURE 7-2   Illustration of hypothesized models of predicted genetic and environmental effects on neurodevelopmental change using twin study designs. Developmental change modeled here is based on a region that demonstrates decreasing volume with age during normal development. See text for detailed explanation. CNTL = control; DZU = dizygotic unaffected; DZA = dizygotic affected; MZA = monozygotic affected; MZU = monozygotic unaffected.

the design and monitoring of treatment interventions. If neurodegenerative changes are in fact present, it would clearly be a goal to prevent this effect with interventions that begin with the expression of an episode of illness. Differences observed prior to the onset of illness would suggest an earlier or preventive treatment strategy.

Family and twin studies are the ideal paradigm for examining neurodevelopmental or neurodegenerative models by providing the ability to study affected individuals and individuals at risk in comparison to related family members who do not develop affective disorders. The inclusion of unrelated control family members is necessary to establish differences from the general population that may not be noted when examining genetically related individuals. Figure 7-2 illustrates how a combination of cross-sectional and longitudinal data from a twin study could clarify developmental versus degenerative changes using monozygotic and dizygotic twins discordant for an illness of interest in comparison to control twins. All four graphs are based on the assumption that a region of interest is manifesting ongoing developmental change over the ages studied and that the region illustrated represents a region in unaffected control subjects, which has decreasing volume over the age range of interest (a common pattern in subcortical structures during childhood and adolescence [Giedd et al. 1996; Reiss et al. 1996]). Graph A illustrates the expected developmental trajectories for a process that was predominantly neurodevelopmental and under early genetic influence. The developmental curve is nearly identical for the monozygotic twins, both affected and unaffected, and is significantly lower than the developmental curve for the control subjects. The affected dizygotic twin is similar to the monozygotic twin pair curve. However, the unaffected dizygotic twin would be intermediate between the control and affected twins because unaffected dizygotic twins would share an average of 50% of their genetic material. Graph B illustrates the expected developmental trajectories in the example of a neurodevelopmental process under early environmental influence. In this graph, the affected monozygotic and dizygotic twins are similar to each other. Because the degree of genetic relatedness is not important in an early unique environmental influence, the unaffected co-twins are both similar to the controls. Graph C is an example of a process under late genetic influence. Initially, all the subjects parallel the same developmental trajectory; however, at some point, the affected subjects deviate from the control curve and the monozygotic co-twins parallel their affected co-twin, whereas the unaffected dizygotic twin would again be intermediate. Finally, Graph D is an example of a developmental process that is under early genetic influence with later additional environmental influence. In this model, both the affected twins and the monozygotic unaffected twins display a developmental deviation early in normal development (as in Graph A). However, when the environmental influence is presented (e.g., certain social stressors, viral illness, or the onset of illness itself), the affected twins begin to deviate from both the at-risk monozygotic twins and the control twins. There are a number of other potential patterns that could be modeled and tested.

Although significant information could be gained from cross-sectional studies with twin pairs, developmental data examining normal neurodevelopment (Giedd et al., 1999) highlighted the need for longitudinal studies of the same subjects to best characterize neurodevelopmental trajectories. Furthermore, Giedd et al. (1999) demonstrated that a number of developmental trends that were apparent in longitudinal study with the same subjects were not apparent or were masked in their earlier cross-sectional study of normal brain development. This effect was largely due to the substantial degree of normal variability present among subjects, which obscures some developmental trends when only cross-sectional data are examined.

Returning to the example of hippocampal volume changes associated with major depression, the author hypothesizes that differences in hippocampal volume will demonstrate neurodegenerative changes and be greater in twins with longer duration of illness than in twin pairs where the duration of illness in the affected twin has been shorter. In this example, the phenotypic description of imaging parameters associated with a disorder will change over time. It is already clear that there are clinical symptom phenotype changes during development and developmental phenotypic changes in neuroendocrine measures associated with mood disorders (Birmaher et al. 1996; Dahl et al. 1992). Developmental changes in imaging parameter phenotype are likely to be present in a number of early-onset disorders. Given that normal developmental progression occurs in many regional brain volumes, we hypothesize that illness processes may interfere or interact with normal developmental processes, thus changing phenotypic description over time. Therefore, some regions may begin similar in size and shape to unaffected children. However, the deviation from normal may become more pronounced as development progresses. Although ongoing developmental change and its effects on phenotypic description imply increased complexity for research and clinical practice, the evidence in support of this complex interactive model is growing. A twin or family study design is a powerful design to specify and characterize this type of model. The pattern of these changes can begin to be established in cross-sectional studies when high-risk family or twin designs are employed (see Figure 7-2). However, longitudinal family or twins studies of affected, high-risk, and control subjects will be important to more precisely characterize these models. Such studies are currently under way in the author's laboratory.

Estimation of Genetic and Environmental Contributions to Imaging Differences

Through the use of a twin design, one can estimate genetic and environmental contributions to structural differences using quantitative genetic analysis techniques. Path analytic modeling, commonly used in twin and family studies, can derive estimates of the relative contribution of environmental and genetic factors to parameters of interest, including quantitative image variables such as structural volumes, shape characteristics, or regional activation. A general example is illustrated in Figure 7-3, which demonstrates how a simple path analysis model could be tested to estimate additive genetic, common environment, and unique environmental contributions to the volume of a region of interest. The goal of these analyses is to determine the amount of the variance in the regional volumes that can be explained by genetic and environmental factors. Such path models can be further specified in a number of ways to estimate shared and specific contributions of factors to a specific variable, such as shared genetic contribution to both depression and a structural volume of interest. A bivariate model, illustrated in Figure 7-4, would estimate the amount of shared additive genetic factors between a disorder of interest such as depression and specific regions such as the subgenual prefrontal cortex (SGPFC). It would also estimate the unique contribution of additive genetic effects to depression alone and SGPFC volume alone. Analogous estimates for both shared environmental influence and unique environmental influence could also be

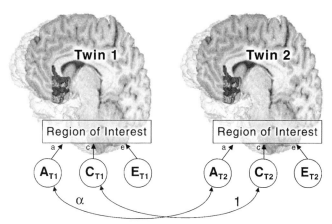

FIGURE 7-3 Simple path model for genetic-environmental contribution to a region of interest. The path diagram illustrated is the general univariate model that could be used to estimate the contribution of additive genetic (a), common environment (c), and unique environmental (e) factors to differences in regional brain volume. The subscripts T1 and T2 refer to measures for variables in twin 1 and twin 2 of a given twin pair. The path coefficient $\alpha = 1$ for monozygotic (MZ) twin pairs and $\alpha = 0.5$ for dizygotic (DZ) twin pairs. The figure illustrates a reconstruction of midline medial prefrontal cortex gyri; the most superior gyrus represents the subgenual prefrontal cortex.

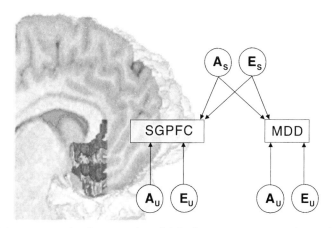

FIGURE 7-4 An example of a general model for bivariate genetic analyses of potential shared influence of genetic and environmental factors on measured variables—the SGPFC and MDD. A_U and E_U represent unique or independent additive genetic or unique environmental effects on the variables of interest. A_X and E_X represent shared additive genetic and shared unique environmental effects between the variables of interest (SGPFC and MDD). The illustration represents the gryus of the medial prefrontal cortex. The most superior gyrus is the subgenual prefrontal cortex.

derived. Models also can be developed and tested to include the increased complexity of changes over time (e.g., characterizing changes in regions over time, and estimating developmental or neurodegenerative changes and the genetic and environmental contributions to those processes).

CONCLUSION

The combination of these two powerful research strategies—neuroimaging and behavioral genetic analyses—has the potential to add substantially to our understanding of affective disorders and how genetic risk confers susceptibility to the onset and progression of affective disorders. Imaging designs can enhance genetic studies by providing information to differentiate heterogeneous disorders, provide quantitative variables to improve linkage analysis studies, and help in understanding the pathophysiologic mechanisms by which genetic risk translates to neuropathology. Conversely, twin and family designs offer a number of advantages for imaging investigations. These advantages comprise the inclusion of better-matched control subjects to improve sensitivity to detect differences associated with disorder and of at-risk subjects to help in distinguishing neurodevelopmental from neurodegenerative mechanisms and to provide for the possibility to estimate genetic and environmental contributions to demonstrated differences through the use of path analytic statistical analysis.

Specifically related to affective disorders, there is evidence for structural brain changes in specific medial and orbital prefrontal cortex, as well as in highly interrelated limbic regions such as the amygdala. Some of these differences have been demonstrated in early-onset depression. It is not yet clear which neuromorphometric differences are present prior to the onset of disorder or which may occur after the onset, or coincident with the onset, of disorder. Regions that are implicated in the pathophysiology of major mood disorders are known to demonstrate ongoing neurodevelopment throughout childhood and adolescence (Giedd et al. 1996). This raises the possibility that the onset of affective disorders during ongoing neurodevelopment may alter the course of normal neurodevelopment, thus leaving the individual more vulnerable to future episodes of illness. We are currently in the process of testing these hypotheses with an epidemiologically ascertained sample of adolescent and young adult women twins with early-onset mood disorders. Furthermore, we are examining the relationship of the genetic risk for affective disorder and the expression of disorder in relation to alterations in brain structure in regions of interest in specific medial-orbital-prefrontal-subcortical limbic circuits. Through the use of a twin design, we are estimating the contribution of environmental and genetic effects to differences in these regions. Using this design, we seek to further refine the characterization of structural differences in related limbic circuit structures to delineate homogeneous endophenotypes associated with now heterogeneous diagnoses of affective disorders.

REFERENCES

Altshuler LL, Bartzokis G, Grieder T, et al: An MRI study of temporal lobe structures in men with bipolar disorder or schizophrenia. Biol Psychiatry 48:147–162, 2000

Birmaher R, Ryan ND, Williamson DE, et al: Childhood and adolescent depression: a review of the past 10 years. Part II. J Am Acad Child Adolesc Psychiatry 35:1575–1583, 1996

Botteron K, Figiel G: The neuromorphometry of affective disorders, in Brain Imaging in Psychiatry. Edited by Krishnan K, Doraiswamy M. New York, Dekker, 1997, pp 145–184

Botteron KN, Raichle ME, Drevets WC, et al: Volumetric reduction in left subgenual prefrontal cortex in early onset depression. Biol Psychiatry, in press

Bremner JD: Does stress damage the brain? Biol Psychiatry 45:797–805, 1999

Bremner JD, Narayan M, Anderson ER, et al: Hippocampal volume reduction in major depression. Am J Psychiatry 157:115–118, 2000

Csernansky JC, Joshi SC, Wang L, et al: Hippocampal morphometry in schizophrenia by high dimensional brain mapping. Proc Natl Acad Sci USA 95:11406–11411, 1998

Dahl RE, Ryan ND, Williamson DE: The regulation of sleep and growth hormone in adolescent depression. J Am Acad Child Adolesc Psychiatry 31:615–621, 1992

Drevets W, Price J, Simpson J, et al: Subgenual prefrontal cortrex abnormalities in mood disorders. Nature 386:824–827, 1997

Drevets WC: Prefrontal cortical-amygdalar metabolism in major depression. Ann NY Acad Sci 877:614–637, 1999

Frangou S, Sharma T, Sigmudsson T, et al: The Maudsley family study: 4 normal planum temporale asymmetry in familial schizophrenia. a volumetric MRI study. Br J Psychiatry 170:328–333, 1997

George MS, Ketter TA, Parekh PI, et al: Blunted left cingulate activation in mood disorder subjects during a response interference task (the Stroop). J Neuropsychiatry Clin Neurosci 9:55–63, 1997

Giedd JN: Normal brain development: ages 4–18, in Brain Imaging in Psychiatry. Edited by Krishnan K, Doraiswamy M, New York, Dekker, 1997, pp 103–120

Giedd JN, Snell JW, Lange N, et al: Quantitative magnetic resonance imaging of human brain development: ages 4–18. Cereb Cortex 6:551–560, 1996

Giedd J, Castellanos F, Rajapakse J, et al: Sexual dimorphism of the developing human brain. Prog Neuropsychopharmacol Biol Psychiatry 21:1185–1201, 1997

Giedd JN, Blumenthal J, Jeffries NO, et al: Brain development during childhood and adolescence: a longitudinal MRI study. Nat Neurosci 2:861, 1999

Hirayasu Y, Shenton ME, Salisbury DF, et al: Subgenual cingulate cortex volume in first-episode psychosis. Am J Psychiatry 156:1091–1093, 1999

Honer WG, Bassett AS, Smith GN, et al: Temporal lobe abnormalities in multigenerational families with schizophrenia. Biol Psychiatry 36:737–743, 1994

Hudziak JJ: Identification of phenotypes for molecular genetic studies of common childhood psychopathology, in Handbook of Psychiatric Genetics. Edited by Blum K, Noble EP. Boca Raton, FL, CRC Press, 1996, pp 201–217

Mayberg HS, Starkstein SE, Sadzot B, et al: Selective hypometabolism in the inferior frontal lobe in depressed patients with Parkinson's disease. Ann Neurol 28:57–64, 1990

Mayberg HS, Starkstein SE, Peyser CE, et al: Paralimbic frontal lobe hypometabolism in depression associated Huntington's disease. Neurology 42:1791–1797, 1992

Mayberg HS, Brannan SK, Mahurin RK, et al: Cingulate function in depression: a potential predictor of treatment response. Neuroreport 8:1057–1061, 1997

Mayberg HS, Liotti M, Brannan SK, et al: Reciporcal limbic-cortical function and negative mood: converging PET findings in depression and normal sadness. Am J Psychiatry 156:675–682, 1999

McCarley RW, Wible CG, Frumin M, et al: MRI anatomy of schizophrenia. Biol Psychiatry 45:1099–1119, 1999

Neuman RJ, Geller B, Rice JP, et al: Increased prevalence and earlier onset of mood disorders among relatives of prepubertal versus adult probands. J Am Acad Child Adolesc Psychiatry 36:466–473, 1997

Öngür D, Drevets W, Price J: Glial reduction in the subgenual prefrontal cortex in mood disorders. Proc Natl Acad Sci USA 95:13290–13295, 1998

Pearlson GD, Barta PE, Powers RE, et al: Medial and superior temporal gyral volumes and cerebral asymmetry in schizophrenia versus bipolar disorder. Biol Psychiatry 41:1–14, 1997

Rajkowska G, Miguel-Hidalgo JJ, Wei J, et al: Morphometric evidence for neuronal and glial prefrontal cell pathology in major depression. Biol Psychiatry 45:1085–1098, 1999

Reiss AL, Abrams MT, Singer HS, et al: Brain development, gender and IQ in children: a volumetric imaging study. Brain 119:1763–1774, 1996

Revely AM, Revely MA, Clifford CA, et al: Cerebral ventricular size in twins discordant for schizophrenia. Lancet I:540–541, 1982

Revely AM, Revely MA, Murray RM: Cerebral ventricular enlargement in non-genetic schizophrenia: a controlled twin study. Br J Psychiatry 144:89–93, 1984

Rice JP: Phenotype definition for genetic studies. Eur Arch Psychiatry Clin Neurosci 243:158–163, 1993

Rice JP, Todorov AA: Stability of diagnosis: application to phenotype definition. Schizophr Bull 20:185–190, 1994

Robins E, Guze SB: Establishment of diagnostic validity in psychiatric illness and its application to schizophrenia. Am J Psychiatry 126:983–987, 1970

Robinson RG: Neuropsychiatric consequences of stroke. Annu Rev Med 48:217–229, 1997

Robinson RG, Boston JD, Starkstein SE, et al: Comparison of mania and depression after brain injury: causal factors. Am J Psychiatry 145:172–178, 1988

Robinson RG, Starkstein SE: Current research in affective disorders following stroke. J Neuropsychiatry Clin Neurosci 2:1–14, 1990

Sackeim HA, Prohovnik I, Moeller JR, et al: Regional cerebral blood flow in mood disorders. Arch Gen Psychiatry 47:60–70, 1990

Sapolsky RM, Krey LC, McEwen BS: The neuorendocrinology of stress and aging: the glucocorticoid cascade hypothesis. Endocr Rev 7:284–301, 1986

Sapolsky RM, Krey LC, McEwen BS: Prolonged glucocorticoid exposure reduces hippocampal neuron number: implications for aging. J Neurosci 5:1222–1227, 1985

Sheline YI, Want PW, Gado MH, et al: Hippocampal atrophy in recurrent major depression. Proc Natl Acad Sci USA 93:3908–3913, 1996

Soares JC, Mann JJ: The anatomy of mood disorders—review of structural neuroimaging studies. Biol Psychiatry 41:86–106, 1997

Staal WG, Hulshoff, Pol HE, et al: Structural brain abnormalities in patients with schizophrenia and their healthy siblings. Am J Psychiatry 157:416–421, 2000

Suddath RL, Christison GW, Torrey EF, et al: Anatomical abnormalities in the brains of monozygotic twins discordant for schizophrenia. N Engl J Med 322:789–794, 1990

Tsuang MT, Faraone SV, Lyons MJ: Identification of the phenotype in psychiatric genetics. Psychiatry Clin Neurosci 243:131–142, 1993

Vakili K, Pillay SS, Lafer B, et al: Hippocampal volume in primary unipolar major depression: a magnetic resonance imaging study. Biol Psychiatry 47:1087–1090, 2000

Weinberger DR, DeLisi LE, Neophytides AN, et al: Familial aspects of CT scan abnormalities in chronic schizophrenic patients. Psychiatry Res 4:65–71, 1981

PART III   LONGITUDINAL STUDIES

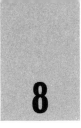

8

Psychopathology and the Life Course

Stephen L. Buka, Sc.D.
Stephen E. Gilman, Sc.D.

The field of "developmental epidemiology" seeks to integrate elements of modern epidemiology (Rothman 1998) and developmental psychology to the scientific investigation of the etiology, course, and treatment of psychiatric disorders (Angold and Costello 1995; Buka and Lipsitt 1994). In this chapter, we explore the implications of overlaying such a developmental perspective onto the task of refining a scientifically based psychiatric nosology for the twenty-first century.

Attempts to classify human mental disorder date back at least 5,000 years (Mack et al. 1994). From the days of Hippocrates, there has been a tension between strictly descriptive/empirical approaches and etiologic/ theory-based classification systems. This tension is reflected in current debates between essentialist and nominalist approaches to define mental disorder (Birley 1990; Clark 1999). Although some researchers contend that "the question of whether certain conditions are disorders or nondisorders has no true scientific answer" (Lilienfeld and Marino 1999, p. 401), in general, the development of an increasingly valid psychiatric nosology has been a long-standing concern in psychiatric research (Kendler 1990; Panzetta 1974; Robins and Guze 1970). The challenge that our field faces is how, with increasing accuracy or validity, to best characterize the various forms of human psychological and psychiatric disorder and dysfunction experienced throughout the life course. That is, in the complicated warp and weave that characterizes the vast variety or heterogeneity of human experience, how do we identify, distinguish, quantify, and possibly categorize relatively homogenous forms of psychopathology? This is, of course, the fundamental first step in our branch of science. Methodologic developments of the past quarter-century, including structured diagnostic interviews and widely disseminated operational definitions, have lead to dramatic advances in the reliability of classification. As Kendell (1989) argued, the issue of reliability has largely been settled, and it is now the challenge of validity that confronts the field of psychiatry.

A key distinction between reliability and validity bears emphasizing. That is, although efforts to produce more reliable classifications operate entirely on the empirical field, at the level of operational criteria, observations, measures, and empirical indicants, validity always involves a two-level process—the first being conceptual and abstract, and the second being empirical and observed (Nunnally 1978). Validity concerns the correspondence between our empirical indicants, our diagnostic criteria and measurement methods, and the constructs and ideas onto which we hope they will map. Reliability is entirely an empirical process, whereas validity forces us to grapple with our fundamental concepts of mental disorder. Thus, as Miettinen (1985) wrote, the first principle in medical science involves specification of the conceptual entity of interest, *followed* by the operationalization of this abstract entity. This process is inherent in all branches of empirical science and medical research, and is particularly challenging in psychiatry, given the abstract nature of our topic of study.

The publication of the modern *Diagnostic and Statistical Manual of Mental Disorders* (DSM-III, DSM-III-R, DSM-IV, and DSM-IV-TR, beginning in 1980) provided a clear initial set of operational criteria or empirical indicants for our field of inquiry and has helped to propel our field into an era of new discovery and communication. Without common empirical metrics, we have no science, no empirically testable hypotheses, and no clear basis for replication. Instead, we have theory with no formal empirical basis, which does not qualify as science. The DSMs represent a critical scientific advance, but not a final one. So what then are the next major steps in the science of the study of psychopathology?

One strategy for describing those aspects of the human condition that we might term as mental disorders involves the dimensions of person, place, and time. The strength of the present condition/manifestational orientation of the DSM centers on the description of the "person"—symptoms experienced by the individual and the resulting consequences for the individual. Descriptions of such symptoms come from years of elegant clinical description of the presenting problems of people seeking or obtaining treatment. Surely work remains to be done to fine-tune person-level elements

for DSM-V (whether five or six symptoms of inattention qualify for a diagnosis attention-deficit disorder [ADD]; which constellation of positive or
negative symptoms qualify for schizophrenia).

However, refinement of these cross-sectional, person-level descriptors
would yield only a marginal advancement to the current nosology and
involve more modifications of person-level symptoms along the lines of the
changes of the past three versions of the DSM. A bolder strategy with greater
potential for scientific growth would come from incorporating some of the
other key dimensions of the human condition to our current nosological
stragegy, not simply modifying the elements already in place.

Much could be said about strategies for incorporating various dimensions of "place"—that is, the setting in which symptoms are expressed, the
relationship of the act and individual to the larger context in which he or
she functions, and cultural variations in norms and behaviors. However,
for the current discussion, we focus on alternatives to further incorporate
the dimension of "time" into the nosology of the twenty-first century.

There are at least three frames relevant for psychiatric nosology: disease
history (or the course of the presenting condition), life history (including
antecedent events that may or may not be part of the presenting syndrome),
and species history, or an evolutionary perspective. Regarding disease history, the concept of time is central to the description of person-level symptom data that are the forte of the DSMs. The DSM is replete with a variety
of temporal descriptors. These descriptors are focused predominantly at
the presenting condition or current disease state and are typically limited
to a relatively short time frame that is bounded by the onset of the "*present*
distress*.*" Examples include the duration of symptoms, which is central to
most diagnoses, and, increasingly, the length of response to pharmacologic
and psychosocial interventions.

The second fashion with which time factors into the discussion of psychopathology draws from the time frame studied by our colleagues, the life
historians (e.g., anthropologists, ethnographers, developmental psychologists). This time frame—the life course—figures heavily in the scholarly
literature on both the causes and conceptualization of major categories
of psychopathology. The need to add a time frame to DSM-II was noted
by Panzetta (1974) and remains a concern in current critiques of DSM-
IV. We, thus, contend that the lifespan time frame figures into the vast
majority of etiologic theory and for the vast majority of psychiatric disorders. That is, whether you are interested in neurodevelopmental theories
of schizophrenia, environmental toxins, ADD, life stress, depression, or the
genetic basis of obsessive-compulsive disorder (OCD), our thinking about
causes and classification uniformly involves ideas and concepts *beyond* the
current disease episode. In our field, this is an implicit nosologic tension

that should be brought to the fore and addressed systematically in future classification systems.

The life course time frame also figures heavily not only in our conceptualization of the major forms of psychopathology but also in most scholarly discussions of the validation of the proposed nosology. In their classic article on the establishment of diagnostic validity in psychiatric illness, Robins and Guze (1970) listed follow-up study (or course following the onset of a disease episode) as one strategy for validating a proposed nosology. Panzetta (1974) went further to propose that we consider course prior to disease onset as a validation strategy.

The third general fashion in which time figures into nosologic reasoning involves a generational or evolutionary time frame. In a discussion of "harmful dysfunction," Wakefield (1992) offered a challenging and provocative intellectual paradigm for conceptualizing and defining psychiatric disorders. Simply stated, Wakefield's concept of harmful dysfunction proposed that mental disorders can be broadly characterized according to a subjective component, harm experienced by the patient, and an objective component, dysfunction. He defined dysfunction as "a failure of some mechanism in the organism to perform its natural function" (p. 383) and that "a natural function of an organ or other mechanism is an effect of the organ or mechanism that enters into an explanation of the existence, structure, or activity of the organ or mechanism" (p. 383). His discussion of what does and does not constitute dysfunction to the human organism provides a useful, although controversial (Lilienfeld and Marino 1999), common language and framework for discussions of the boundaries of mental disorder. It also forces us to consider human functioning from an evolutionary time frame, reminiscent of the postulate of Piaget that the adaptive and normative development of the individual (ontology) has parallels in the adaptive development of the species (phylogeny).

This discussion of the various manners in which time figures into our conceptualization and operationalization of psychiatric disorders raises a larger point about the relevance of the study of human development to psychiatric nosology and research. In large part, most writings that called for increased adoption of a developmental perspective into psychiatric research have focused on the fact that children and adolescents are not "miniature adults," rallied for increased recognition of biological and emotional maturation of children and adolescents, and urged that this be reflected in age-appropriate diagnostic criteria and procedures. We would go further than this and argue that elements of life course human development are central to the valid classification of most forms of psychopathology in both childhood and adulthood. As Rutter (1989) stated: "Homo sapiens is a social animal and social development and function can only be understood in relation to a person's interactions and transactions with his/her social environment" (p. 25). Current thinking about lifespan development is concerned with "dynamic notions of the continuing interplay over time between intrinsic (e.g., genetic) and extrinsic influences on individual normal and abnormal development" (p. 24). The following list indicates some of the features of current lifespan developmental theory that distinguish the life course orientation from earlier orientations of child development theory and that have implications for the classification and study of psychiatric disorder:

1. Longitudinal perspective across the life course
2. Heterotypic/homotypic continuity
3. Individual differences in response to transitions
4. Biosocial orientation—intrinsic/extrinsic influences
5. Interaction of risk and protective factors
6. Niche picking—effects of behavior (and genes) on context

However, returning to the introductory theme, our key argument is that, in our goal to generate increasingly valid and useful psychiatric classification systems that attempt to fit a conceptual and empirical framework to the complex processes and phenomena of people's lives, behaviors, thoughts, and emotions, one central pillar of a scientific agenda for the twenty-first century should be the careful and considered, but considerable investment of scientific resources, intellectual, and material, into the study of time.

So what, then, is the state of the art for our current psychiatric nosology with respect to the dimension of time? We reviewed DSM-IV for the various uses of time in current diagnostic nosology. The two most common applications pertain to symptom duration and syndrome duration. For instance, a prespecified length of symptom duration is required for many disorders, such as attention-deficit/hyperactivity disorder (ADHD: symptoms of at least 6 months' duration), panic disorder (e.g., persistent concern of at least 1 month's duration), and major depressive disorder (MDD; symptoms of at least 2 weeks' duration). Furthermore, certain diagnoses require that the symptom cluster or syndrome persist for a certain interval to reach diagnostic criteria. Such examples would be schizophrenia, which requires continuous signs of the disturbance for at least 6 months, or dysthymic disorder.

Table 8-1 summarizes other, less common applications of time in diagnostic criteria in DSM-IV. Certain diagnoses specify a maximum age at onset. For instance, in ADHD symptoms must have an onset prior to age 7, and in somatization disorder symptoms must have an onset by age 30. Information on the course of disorder (subsequent to disorder onset) is used to distinguish single from recurrent major depression. Similarly, information on the duration of disorder (subsequent to onset) distinguishes

TABLE 8-1 Applications of time in DSM-IV diagnostic criteria

	Diagnostic criteria	Subtyping
Age at onset	ADHD Somatization disorder	Dysthymia (early/late)
Course of disorder	Depression (single/recurrent)	Substance dependence (course specifiers)
Duration	Schizophreniform/schizophrenia Dysthymia/major depression	PTSD (acute/chronic) Pain disorder (acute/chronic)
Pattern	Bipolar disorders	Bipolar disorders
Antecedent event	PTSD	Delirium/dementia

Note. ADHD = attention-deficit/hyperactivity disorder; PTSD = posttraumatic stress disorder.

major diagnoses such as schizophrenia from schizophreniform disorder and depression from dysthymic disorder. The pattern, rather than the duration, of disorder is used to diagnose bipolar disorder as distinct from manic episodes. Finally, posttraumatic stress disorder (PTSD) is the well-recognized sole instance in which occurrence of an antecedent event (of presumed etiologic significance) is a formal criterion for diagnosis.

All the temporal features that are used as diagnostic criteria for the major Axis I disorders (onset, duration, pattern, and course of symptoms) are also used to distinguish subtypes within diagnostic group. As shown in Table 8-1, information on age at onset is used to diagnose subtypes of dysthymia, namely early onset (prior to age 21) and late onset. For the substance-related disorders, a number of subtypes exist, distinguished by disorder course (e.g., early full remission, early partial remission, sustained partial remission). Syndrome duration is used to subtype PTSD and pain disorders into acute and chronic forms. Related to this is the strategy used to distinguish subtypes of mood disorders, in particular, bipolar disorder, in terms of the full pattern rather than simply the duration of the disorder, such as diagnoses with and without interepisode recovery, seasonal pattern, and rapid cycling. Finally, there are many instances in which subtypes are distinguished by the presence/absence of an antecedent condition, such as the various forms of dementia and mental disorders occurring secondary to a general medical condition.

The point of this brief review is that temporal features both antecedent and subsequent to symptom onset are used throughout DSM-IV, both as primary diagnostic criteria and to distinguish clinically meaningful subtypes. However, these various dimensions of time and course are applied unevenly through our current taxonomic system. One useful strategy to reduce the heterogeneity within DSM-IV diagnoses is to encourage the proliferation of subtypes within major diagnostic categories, through a more extensive and even application of these temporal aspects, including those that occur prior to the onset of the full presenting syndrome. Such a strategy is, of course, largely beyond the capacity of most clinical researchers, whose life history information is obtained at the time of clinical presentation. However, strategies for gaining life history information (McHugh and Slavney 1998) through clinical interview methods are a core feature of clinical diagnosis. The growing number of prospective community-based samples should also yield critical information on this topic. Although beyond the scope of the current discussion, efforts to subtype major diagnostic categories by prodromal features (Eaton et al. 1995; Fava and Kellner 1991; Murphy et al. 1989; Yung 1996), age at onset, and patterns of recurrence (Angst and Merikangas 1997) offer promise.

Accordingly, we have three recommendations for defining psychopathology in the twenty-first century that are mindful of the tension in our field between the need for a taxonomic system that is clinically useful and the need for one that possesses scientific utility. The first proposal is to take an essentialist, or largely rational/conceptual position, in the description and definition of the major diagnostic entities. Currently, there are fewer than 20 major classes of mental disorders described in DSM-IV (e.g., mood disorders, psychotic disorders, substance-related disorders). These have real-world utility for clinician and patient alike and may suffice for many non-research-oriented consumers of our classification system. Our second proposal is that to continue to propel scientific discovery in our field, successive refinements of our nosologic systems should be systematic and planful in new additions. Again, additions or overlays to the basic diagnostic categories should be conceptually, more than empirically, motivated. Such a step (with a resulting propulsion of discovery in the field) occurred in 1980 with the publication of DSM-III and the conceptual commitment to both define what constituted "mental disorder" and to adopt a largely atheoretical strategy in the formulation of diagnostic types and subtypes (Spitzer 1999). This represented a major conceptual leap forward from previous classification systems; subsequent revisions (DSM-III-R and DSM-IV) have been empirical variations on this conceptual theme but have not systematically introduced new encompassing conceptual themes. Examples of new themes that could be used to refine and subtype the major diagnostic entities in future classification systems include moving from the current manifestational, cross-sectional, patient-level orientation to systems that highlight 1) alternative overarching definitions of mental disorder, such as the harmful dysfunction analysis (Wakefield 1999); 2) heightened attention to the role of context and setting in symptom expression; 3) comorbidity; and/or 4) the current discussion of focusing on temporal and life course aspects of symptom and syndromal occurrence.

Finally, our third proposal is that these systematic and successive introductions of new themes around which to order the classification of mental disorders be largely applied through the identification and refinement of *subtypes* of disorders. Although we have suggested that the highest order of differentiation of disorders into the major diagnostic categories be based largely on conceptual ideas of the basic essences or forms of mental disorder that naturally occur (and are universal throughout the species), we also propose that alternative strategies for generating subtypes be largely empirically based. We encourage the authors of future DSMs to permit the number of diagnostic subtypes to increase, ideally through the application of some orderly conceptual principles such as those proposed above. An initial step on this path would be to specify subtypes based on the temporal life course dimensions described above. That is, subtype more uniformly, based on age of onset, symptom and syndrome duration and pattern, and prodromal or antecedent conditions.

In Figure 8-1, in schematic form, we summarize the various forms of temporal subtypes that are used in DSM-IV and that we propose be expanded upon in future DSMs. As shown, many current diagnostic subtypes are distinguished by temporal aspects of the disorder. Again, the more

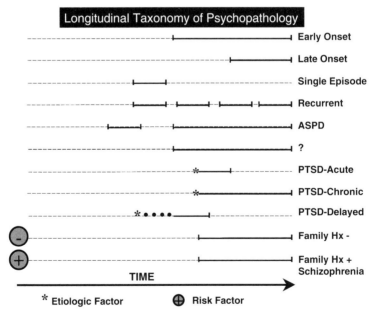

FIGURE 8-1 Schematic depiction of temporally defined diagnostic types and subtypes in DSM-IV. ASPD = antisocial personality disorder; Hx = history; PTSD = posttraumatic stress disorder.

familiar examples include the distinction between early- and late-onset dysthymia, and single episode versus recurrent depression. Several diagnoses that require information about conditions existing prior to the presenting syndrome are also incorporated. We have discussed the novel instance of PTSD, which requires a presumed etiologic event to meet diagnostic criteria and for which there are temporally based subtypes, depending on both symptom duration and the latent phase between qualifying event and syndrome expression. Antisocial personality disorder is another interesting variation on the temporal theme. Here, to meet full diagnostic criteria, in addition to the key criterion of a pattern of antisocial symptoms occurring since age 15, there is a requirement of related behaviors (conduct disorder) with onset before age 15. No diagnostic label exists for those with adult-onset antisocial symptoms. Finally, depicted in Figure 8-1 and as discussed, we contend that with growing etiologic information subclassifications be based on antecedent conditions of presumed etiologic relevance, such as family history of disorder, genetic liability, or exposure to psychosocial stressors.

Some critics have argued that such increases in the number of diagnostic categories and subcategories is a step backward and not forward in the scientific growth of our field. For example, Follette and Houts (1996) noted that from DSM-III to DSM-IV the number of diagnoses grew by approximately 40%. They suggested that "the proliferation of diagnostic categories observed over succeeding editions of the DSM is not consistent with a traditional model of scientific progress" (p. 1125). We side with Wakefield's response to this assertion—that the goal of science is to get the categories right (validity), not simply to obtain the lowest number. At this point in our field, where we have produced reliable but not necessarily valid diagnostic categories, we argue that scientific growth would follow from the introduction and use of both well-reasoned and empirically based diagnostic distinctions. In other words, we propose that for the higher-order general classes of mental disorder we be conceptual "lumpers," but within classes we should be empirical "splitters." Applications of prespecified subtypes include 1) publishing descriptive statistics for these smaller diagnostic subtypes, 2) stratification for clinical trials, and 3) clinical communication and case vignettes. As MacMahon and Pugh (1970) stated, "even in the absence of identification of direct causal factors, epidemiologic criteria may be used to classify or subclassify groups of persons with particular manifestational diseases" (p. 53). At a minimum, we could immediately begin to distinguish family history positive/family history negative subtypes for most major diagnoses. This would incorporate what we have learned about the familial basis of many disorders, reduce diagnostic heterogeneity, and intensify the potential to identify those etiologic factors that may be unique to the nonfamilial subset. Many other educated subtypes can be proposed along the lines described above. We suggest that these subtypes be incorporated into subsequent DSMs and used in our research. However, validation criteria will need to be developed and applied to new diagnostic subtypes prior to their integration into clinical practice.

A primary objective of our recommendations is to disentangle the complex web of influences—and causes—of mental illness. Our underlying assumption—and expectation—is that the identification of etiologic factors be reflected in subsequent diagnostic schema. Since the 1970s, much of the discussion of the process surrounding the refinement of nosologic systems has involved validation. The basic model is that alternative classification strategies should be compared on such key features as results from laboratory studies (biological markers), prognosis, heritability, and response to treatment (Kendell 1989; Robins and Guze 1970). In this view, there is an iterative process in which the adequacy of a classification system is evaluated through these validation strategies, which in turn refines the classification system, and so on. But there is another iterative process set into motion with this approach in which increasingly valid taxonomies spawn new information about the etiology of disorder. As our diagnostic entities gain in reliability and validity, we are forced to consider how to incorporate the resulting growth in knowledge about etiology for these conditions.

This harkens back to a familiar criticism of the DSMs that have also been discussed in detail by others. Namely, the firm position taken with DSM-III that these classification systems should be "atheoretical" (Follette and Houts 1996), and language included in the introduction of DSM-III and DSM-III-R where

> The approach taken in DSM-III is atheoretical with regard to etiology or pathophysiological process except for those disorders where this is well established and therefore included in the definition of the disorder.... The major justification for this generally atheoretical approach taken in DSM-III with regard to etiology is that the inclusion of etiological variables would be an obstacle to use of the manual by clinicians of varying theoretical orientations, since it would not be possible to present all reasonable etiological theories for each disorder. (American Psychiatric Association, 1980, p. 7; 1987, p. xxiii)

In their classic text on epidemiology, MacMahon and Pugh (1970) distinguished between two distinct strategies to categorize disease entities— manifestational criteria and causal criteria. As discussed in this text, there are arguments both for and against classifying diseases and disorders on the basis of manifestational criteria, causal criteria, or some combination of each (MacMahon and Pugh 1970). In the absence of knowledge of causal factors for a disorder, manifestational criteria provide the only alternative for classification. However, as causal factors are identified, these manifestational criteria are either discarded or revised to define new disease entities. As MacMahon and Pugh noted, "The results of a successful study may reveal causal criteria around which revised groupings of ill persons could be made. Thus, disease classification is not only a prerequisite of epidemiologic study but also one of its goals" (p. 52).

To be evenhanded, it may have been desirable for the early DSMs to have been atheoretical and not favor one theoretical orientation over another. As a result, the modern DSMs have generally tended to be nonetiologic with regard to nosology (with the exception of PTSD) and have adopted a purely manifestational classification strategy. However, in an attempt to be theory neutral, it would be scientifically regressive for the DSMs to be etiologically neutral and ignore growing scientific evidence of causality in successive refinements of the classification scheme. Despite the strict "atheoretical" language of the DSMs, there are instances of causal criteria used in this classification system (e.g., PTSD, substance-induced psychoses, cognitive disorders due to medical conditions).

The strong emphasis on manifestational criteria in the recent DSMs is a solid foundation of future inquiry into the etiology of psychiatric disorders. In an iterative fashion, diagnostic boundaries will be refined and valid entities will be identified. Also in an iterative fashion, manifestational criteria will need to give way to criteria based on etiologic factors. Future DSMs may be atheoretical, or better, theory neutral, but they should not be nonetiologic.

Fava and Kellner (1991) noted that

> the operational definitions of DSM give only a flat, two-dimensional view of the patient's illness because they ignore features that earlier clinicians put much weight upon, such as family history, previous episodes and responses to previous treatments. The study of infectious disease, in its symptomatic subdivision among prodromal, acute, subacute and residual phases provides at least a warning against undue restrictions of explorations of the dynamic assessment of the patient, which includes biography. (p. 828)

We contend that this warning has relevance to both the clinician and the scientist consumer of the current and future DSMs. Systematically incorporating information about the life course into both the major diagnostic categories and subtypes is a much-needed enhancement that should yield dramatic increases in scientific growth for the next generation of research in mental disorders. Introduction of the atheoretical, person-oriented, manifestational orientation of DSM-III, DSM-III-R, and DSM-IV resulted in an initial burst of new scientific discovery. As a field, we must now reap the harvest of this fruitful period of psychiatric research toward a new classification system that will more thoroughly incorporate information on course and etiology in the diagnostic criteria for the twenty-first century.

REFERENCES

American Psychiatric Association: Diagnostic and Statistical Manual of Mental Disorders, 3rd Edition (DSM-III). Washington, DC, American Psychiatric Association, 1980

American Psychiatric Association: Diagnostic and Statistical Manual of Mental Disorders, 3rd Edition, Revised (DSM-III-R). Washington, DC, American Psychiatric Association, 1987

American Psychiatric Association: Diagnostic and Statistical Manual of Mental Disorders, 4th Edition (DSM-IV). Washington, DC, American Psychiatric Association, 1994

American Psychiatric Association: Diagnostic and Statistical Manual of Mental Disorders, 4th Edition, Text Revision (DSM-IV-TR). Washington, DC, American Psychiatric Association, 2000

Angold A, Costello EJ: Developmental epidemiology. Epidemiol Rev 17:74–82, 1995

Angst J, Merikangas K: The depressive spectrum: diagnostic classification and course. J Affect Disord 45:31–40, 1997

Birley JLT: DSM-III: from left to right or from right to left? Br J Psychiatry 157:116–118, 1990

Buka SL, Lipsitt LP: Toward a developmental epidemiology, in Developmental Follow-Up: Concepts, Domains and Methods. Edited by Friedman SL, Haywood HC. San Diego, CA, Academic Press, 1994, pp 331–350

Clark L: Introduction to the special section on the concept of disorder. J Abnorm Psychol 108:371–373, 1999

Eaton WW, Badawi M, Melton B: Prodromes and precursors: epidemiologic data for primary prevention of disorders with slow onset. Am J Psychiatry 152:967–972, 1995

Fava GA, Kellner R: Prodromal symptoms in affective disorders. Am J Psychiatry 148:823–830, 1991

Follette WC, Houts AC: Models of scientific progress and the role of theory in taxonomy development: a case study of the DSM. J Consult Clin Psychol 64:1120–1132, 1996

Kendell RE: Clinical validity. Psychol Med 19:45–55, 1989

Kendler KS: Toward a scientific psychiatric nosology. Arch Gen Psychiatry 47:969–973, 1990

Lilienfeld SO, Marino L: Essentialism revisited: evolutionary theory and the concept of mental disorder. J Abnorm Psychol 108:400–411, 1999

Mack AH FL, Brown R, Frances A: A brief history of psychiatric classification. Psychiatric Clin N Am 17:515–522, 1994

MacMahon B, Pugh TF: Epidemiology: Principles and Methods. Boston, MA, Little, Brown, 1970

McHugh PR, Slavney PR: The Perspectives of Psychiatry. Baltimore, MD, Johns Hopkins University Press, 1998

Miettinen OS: Theoretical Epidemiology: Principles of Occurrence Research in Medicine. New York, Wiley, 1985

Murphy JM, Sobol AM, Olivier DC, et al: Prodromes of depression and anxiety: the Stirling County study. Br J Psychiatry 155:490–495, 1989

Nunnally JC: Psychometric Theory. New York, McGraw-Hill, 1978

Panzetta AF: Toward a scientific psychiatric nosology. Arch Gen Psychiatry 30:154–161, 1974

Robins E, Guze SB: Establishment of diagnostic validity in psychiatric illness: its application to schizophrenia. Am J Psychiatry 126:107–111, 1970

Rothman KJ: Modern Epidemiology. Philadelphia, PA, Lippincott-Raven, 1998

Rutter M: Pathways from childhood to adult life. J Child Psychol Psychiatry 30:23–51, 1989

Spitzer RL: Harmful dysfunction and the DSM definition of mental disorder. J Abnorm Psychol 108:430–432, 1999

Wakefield JC: The concept of mental disorder: on the boundary between biological facts and social values. Am Psychologist 47:373–388, 1992

Yung AR: The prodromal phase of first-episode psychosis: past and current conceptualizations. Schizophr Bull 22:353–370, 1996

9

Detecting Longitudinal Patterns of Alcohol Use

John E. Helzer, M.D.
John S. Searles, Ph.D.

Concerns about the adequacy of the current nosological model for psychopathology are highlighted in the study of alcoholism, in which it seems inescapable that attempts to define alcohol abuse and dependence have left researchers with a heterogeneous set of disorders. A categorical taxonomy continues to be highly utilitarian for decision making in clinical settings. However, a relatively simple definitional system, such as DSM-IV (American Psychiatric Association 1994), which defines classes that are likely heterogeneous, may be problematic for other uses, such as genetics research. In the latter context, the need is for a more subtle, multifaceted typology that minimizes or even eliminates phenotypic heterogeneity relative to genotypes. An empirically based, dimensional classification might serve these needs. As cumbersome as it might be for clinical use, there are potentially significant research advantages in a dimensional system that uses differential scores on several parameters simultaneously, is heavily empirical, and can only be successfully applied by computer.

This work was supported by a grant from the National Institutes of Alcohol Abuse and Addiction: AA 1954 (Dr. Helzer).

One dimension that might be useful in the taxonomy of alcoholism is consumption patterns. Until now, consumption data, as they exist in the typical study, would probably not be adequate for taxonomy. In most epidemiological and even clinical research, the characterizations of drinking patterns vary widely, and most studies rely on only one or two items to establish what then gets labeled a pattern (Epstein et al. 1995). Furthermore, the inquiry is generally retrospective over long periods of time.

Although there is considerable agreement as to the importance of improving the ways in which drinking patterns are measured, it is unclear what methodology should be used to accomplish this. Retrospective measurement is particularly problematic, as is illustrated below. However, emerging measurement technologies are beginning to make continuous, prospective collection of consumption and other daily data a reality. Assessments that do not involve face-to-face interaction with an interviewer, often called ecological assessments, may prove useful.

A method we are currently using in our research group called Interactive Voice Response (IVR) is an example of an ecological assessment (Mundt et al. 1995; Searles et al. 1995, 2000). IVR is essentially a method for interaction between an individual and a computer through the medium of a telephone using the touch-tone keypad. Typically, an automated script poses questions following a branching logic format, and the caller keys in responses. IVR is familiar primarily because of its commercial applications and can be frustrating when the caller's needs are not met, which of course is sometimes the goal. However, several investigators have now applied IVR systems in more responsive ways to enhance clinical efforts of various kinds, including data collection, diagnosis, and follow-up facilitation, and have achieved high levels of caller satisfaction. You can even file your federal income tax using an IVR system. Nonetheless, caller satisfaction is variable.

We began our own work in ecological assessment by testing a variety of methods, including telephone answering machines, for daily routine data collection. We settled on an IVR system because of several inherent advantages. First, the touch-tone telephone is familiar, convenient, and ubiquitous, even in rural Vermont. Second, an IVR can easily handle a complex branching script and make this complexity transparent to the caller. Third, entry of clean data is instantaneous, producing a cumulative database that is immediately available. In fact, the caller's own data record can be queried and used to help determine question flow even within a single call.

The 33 subjects for our study shown herein were recruited from participants in another research project that was coming to an end. Originally, the subjects had been recruited from bars and were involved in a study of the psychobiology of alcohol tolerance (Mundt et al. 1997). Fifty subjects from the tolerance study enrolled to participate in this pilot test of using an IVR to collect daily data for a 7-month period. At the end of 7 months, we had additional pilot funds and invited all 50 to continue calling if they wanted; 33 elected to do so. There was no difference in call frequency for the first 7 months among those who elected to continue and the 17 who elected to stop. We terminated this IVR pilot study after 2 years, but many of the 33 subjects had become so accustomed to calling every day that they were disappointed to see the trial come to an end. There were no dropouts during the 7-month phase and only two in the 2-year phase of the study (both at 22 months).

Participants called the IVR system via a toll-free phone number (active throughout the continental United States and Canada) once per day to report their alcohol consumption and other parameters such as mood, level of stress, urge to drink if they had not taken a drink, and so on. We paid them $0.50 per call and also gave them cumulative bonus points that they could periodically exchange for money. If they missed a call, then they would lose some bonus points; however, they could make up most of these points by even more consistent calling. If they called every day without fail, then their payments amounted to about $13.00 per week. With some practice, each call lasted about 2 minutes. The subjects quickly got in the habit of calling religiously and rarely missed a call, even when out of town or on vacation. We continued the calling for 2 full years. In total, for the 33 subjects there were 24,834 possible calls over the 2-year period. As shown below, the subjects completed the vast majority of these calls.

Table 9-1 shows demographic characteristics of the 33 subjects, two-thirds of whom met DSM-IV criteria for alcohol abuse/dependence as ascertained by the Composite International Diagnostic Interview/Substance Abuse Module (CIDI/SAM; Robins et al. 1995) at the index examination.

Table 9-2 shows the questions of the IVR script we used. Once callers identified themselves by keying in their ID number and a unique password, the script began with three questions about the amount of alcohol

TABLE 9-1   Demographics by lifetime diagnostic status

	None ($n = 11$)	Abuse/dependence ($n = 22$)
Age (SD)	36.2 (3.8)	30.4 (1.5)
Education in years (SD)	14.1 (0.81)	13.6 (0.46)
Race (% caucasian)	100	95.5
Marital status (% single)	54.5	63.6
% Employed	81.8	81.8

TABLE 9-2 Interactive voice response script for daily monitoring

1. **BEER:** How many beers did you drink yesterday?
2. **LIQUOR:** How many drinks containing liquor did you have yesterday?
3. **WINE:** How many glasses of wine did you drink yesterday?

IF RESPONSE TO 1, 2, **OR** 3 IS GREATER THAN 0 THEN:

IF RESPONSE TO 1, 2, **AND** 3 IS 0 THEN:

4. **INTOXICATION:** Rate your highest level of intoxication yesterday on a scale of 0 to 10, with 0 being perfectly sober and 10 being as drunk as you've ever been.

5. **DRIVING:** Rate your highest level of intoxication while driving yesterday, from 0 perfectly sober to 10 as drunk as you've ever been. Press 99 if you did not drive yesterday after having 1 or more drinks.

6. **PROBLEMS:** Rate the seriousness of any problems you had because of your drinking yesterday, from 0 no problems to 10 extremely serious problems.

7. **LOCATION:** For the following locations, press 1 if you had at least 1 drink there yesterday and 0 if you didn't:
   a. Home
   b. Friend's
   c. Bar
   d. Restaurant
   e. Vehicle
   f. Work
   g. Somewhere else

4. **URGE:** Rate your urge to drink yesterday on a scale of 0 to 10, with 0 being no urge to drink, and 10 being the strongest urge ever to drink.

5. **HANGOVER:** Rate any hangover you may have had yesterday, from 0 no hangover to 10 the worst hangover you ever had.

6. **REASONS FOR NOT DRINKING YESTERDAY:** For each of the following statements, press 1 if true or 0 if false:
   a. **AVOIDANCE:** I avoided drinking on purpose.
   b. **MONEY:** I couldn't afford to drink.
   c. **ILLNESS:** I didn't feel well.
   d. **OPPORTUNITY:** I had no opportunity to drink.
   e. **MEDICATION:** I was taking a medication.
   f. **SOCIAL INFLUENCE:** The situation I was in discouraged drinking.
   g. **SOMETHING ELSE:** There is another reason I didn't drink yesterday.

8. **CIGARETTES:** How many cigarettes did you smoke yesterday?

9. **STRESS:** Rate your highest level of stress yesterday, on a scale of 0 to 10 with 0 being no stress and 10 being the highest stress you've ever experienced.

10. **ANGER:** Rate your highest level of anger yesterday, from 0 not at all angry to 10 the angriest you've ever been.

11. **SAD:** At your worst, how sad or blue did you feel yesterday, from 0 not at all sad or blue to 10 the saddest you've ever been?

(continued)

TABLE 9-2   Interactive voice response script for daily monitoring *(continued)*

12. **HAPPY:** At your best, how happy did you feel yesterday, from 0 not at all happy to 10 the happiest you've ever been?

13. **RATE YOUR DAY:** Rate yesterday overall from 0 your worst day ever to 10 the best day you've ever had?

14. **HEALTH:** How did you feel physically yesterday, from 0 the sickest you've ever felt to 10 feeling your healthiest?

15. **RELATIONSHIP:** Overall, how well did you get along with your partner yesterday, from 0 the worst it's ever been to 10 the best it's ever been? Press 88 if you did not have any contact with your partner yesterday. Press 99 if you are not currently in a relationship.

16. **PARTNER DRINKING:** How many alcohol drinks did your partner have yesterday?

17. **HOURS WORKED:** How many hours did you work for pay yesterday?

18. **CURRENT INTOXICATION:** How intoxicated do you feel right now, from 0 perfectly sober to 10 as drunk as you've ever been?

---

consumed "yesterday." Because calls could be made at any time day or night, we asked about the previous day to provide a consistent time frame. The script then divided into one branch for those who consumed any alcohol and a separate branch for those who consumed no alcohol in that 24-hour period. The any- and no-consumption branches were of approximately equal length so callers were not motivated to falsely report no consumption just to shorten the interview. In the drinking branch, subjects were asked to rate their highest level of intoxication overall, highest level while driving, and severity of any problems related to alcohol for the reporting period. This was followed by a series of dichotomous questions about drinking locations. Those on the no-consumption branch were asked to rate the strength of their urge to drink, the severity of any hangover, and then a series of dichotomous questions about reasons they did not drink for that reporting period. In the final branch, both groups were asked the number of cigarettes they consumed that day and to rate the items shown on Table 9-2. Each question began with a "keyword" (shown in bold on the table). Questionnaire items could be answered as soon as the caller heard the keyword, greatly shortening the call duration for experienced callers. Each call concluded with an updated account of the subject's balance of dollars and bonus points.

We designed the payment scheme to be behaviorally compelling. Figure 9-1 shows our level of success. During the 2 years of the study, 91.7%

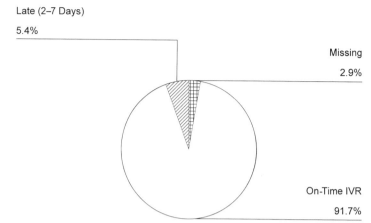

FIGURE 9-1   IVR call rates over a 2-year period.

of the nearly 25,000 calls were made to the IVR system on the appointed day. If there were any missing calls, the IVR reminded the subject of these the next time he or she called. Tardy reports could be made at any time and were accepted as late calls up to 7 days, after which they were pooled with calls that were missing altogether. Adding the on-time and late calls, we received a total of 97%.

Figure 9-2 provides an overview of the weekly consumption in this sample and shows a pattern consistent with expectations. There is more drinking on the weekends, although Sunday is not quite as high as Friday

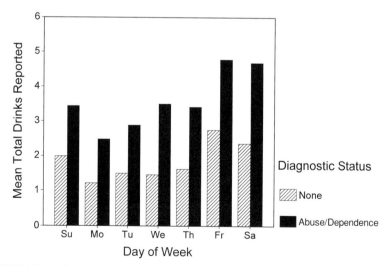

FIGURE 9-2   Daily consumption by diagnostic status.

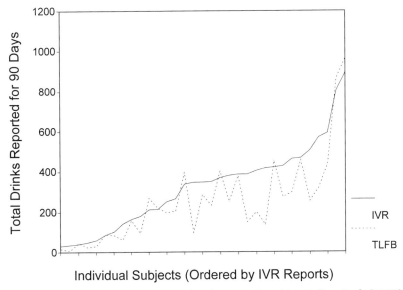

FIGURE 9-3 Interactive Voice Response (IVR) versus Time-Line Follow-Back (TLFB) retrospective for 90 days.

and Saturday. Mean number of drinks is lowest for Monday. The quantities differ between those with and without an alcohol diagnosis, but the pattern is similar. There was also an expected increase in alcohol consumption during holidays, especially for particular holidays, with New Year's Eve and Labor Day showing the largest number of mean drinks for the year.

Figure 9-3 highlights a long-standing concern about retrospective quantification of alcohol consumption. In addition to asking subjects to call the IVR daily, we also performed quarterly face-to-face interviews with the 33 participants during this 2-year study. As part of the quarterly examination, we used the Time-Line Follow-Back (TLFB; Sobell and Sobell 1992) during the first year to obtain retrospective reports of drinking. The TLFB is the current standard for retrospective reports of daily alcohol consumption. It is essentially a calendar; that is, the interviewer helps the respondent fill in landmark dates to serve as mnemonics for a retrospective day-by-day recall of consumption over the period of interest. The TLFB has been used to ascertain retrospective reports for varying periods of time, even throughout a person's lifetime in the most grandiose efforts. Typically, it is used to cover periods of up to several months. In Figure 9-3, subjects are arrayed along the x-axis according to their IVR consumption reports over the 90 days since the last interview. Consumption at the IVR intersect is equivalent to an average of about 1 drink per day at the left extreme of the graph and an average of about 10 drinks per day at the right extreme. The graph shows the comparison between the concurrent IVR reports and the retrospective TLFB reports for the same 90-day period.

Several things are apparent in this comparison. First, there is substantial disagreement between the concurrent and retrospective measures. Second, there is more agreement at the extremes than in the middle of the consumption range. Perhaps those at either extreme are more consistent drinkers. Third, most of the discrepancy, and nearly all the substantial discrepancy, is due to comparative underreporting on the TLFB. We have evidence from informant data in this study and from a previous validity study that subjects' IVR reports are an accurate reflection of their actual daily consumption (Perrine et al. 1995). Therefore, it is reasonable to assume that these discrepancies represent true underreporting on the TLFB rather than overreporting on the IVR. If so, this retrospective underreporting occurred despite the potential rehearsal of the daily IVR phone reports of consumption during the same 90-day period.

Finally, a minority of subjects even in the midrange of reporting shows close agreement between the TLFB and the IVR. We are attempting to find variables that might help to prospectively classify subjects as to level of retrospective accuracy, but we have not been successful so far. If such prediction was successful, it might enable us to construct a metric to correct for retrospective underreporting across an entire sample. This would be highly desirable because most consumption reports in both clinical and research settings are necessarily retrospective.

Next, we began to explore how these consumption results might be used to subclassify drinkers. Figure 9-4 illustrates our attempt to replicate

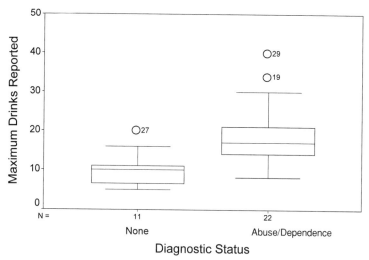

FIGURE 9-4   Maximum drinks reported in a single day by alcohol diagnosis.

a finding by Saccone et al. (2000). In an analysis of data from the Collaborative Study on the Genetics of Alcoholism (COGA), Saccone and her colleagues found that the maximum reported drinks ever consumed in a 24-hour period might be a useful phenotype. It was closely related to a diagnosis of alcoholism in the COGA data. Furthermore, maximum drinks proved to be a quantitative measure to grade nonalcoholic individuals. Figure 9-4 illustrates our similar findings regarding diagnostic discrimination in our 11 subjects without an alcohol diagnosis versus the 22 subjects with an alcohol diagnosis. The boxes show the 25th to the 75th percentile in the maximum drinks reported in any 24-hour period. Overlap is seen only at the extremes of the consumption distribution and outliers (open circles).

To test maximum 24-hour consumption as a quantitative method of subdividing nondiagnosed subjects, we looked at its predictive validity. We correlated maximum drinks reported on the IVR in the first 6-month period of our study with total consumption reported in the next three 6-month periods. Nonalcoholic individuals showed a positive and significant correlation in each period and the correlations were actually highest in the final 6 months. In the alcoholic group, there were no significant correlations, which is also consistent with Saccone et al.'s findings.

We found an interesting relationship between mood and consumption by diagnostic status. In Figure 9-5, mood is the dependent variable and is displayed on a scale standardized across the entire sample on both drinking and nondrinking days, with a mean of 0 and SD of 1. There is a clear difference between the diagnosed and nondiagnosed in terms of the

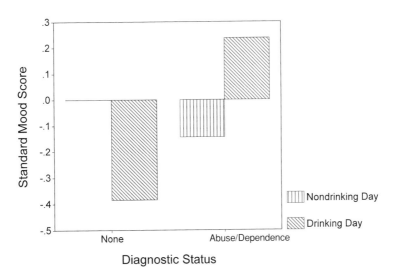

FIGURE 9-5   Mood rating, consumption, and diagnostic status.

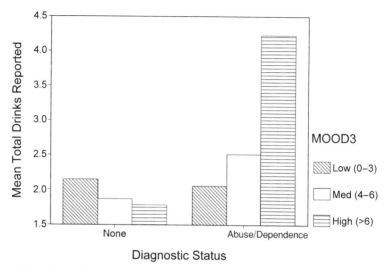

FIGURE 9-6   Alcohol consumption and mood by diagnosis.

mood/consumption relationship. Among those with no diagnosis, mood is right at the mean on nondrinking days, whereas drinking days are associated with significantly lower mood. Those with alcohol abuse/dependence show the opposite relationship. Mood is low on nondrinking days and drinking days are associated with a significantly elevated mood. Because the mood and consumption reports on the IVR are for the same 24-hour period, we are unable to address direction of effect. We plan to examine lagged effects to see if this could be informative as to temporal relations.

Figure 9-6 shows a dose response in the differential relationship between mood and consumption by diagnosis. Mean drinks per 24 hours is somewhat higher on days when mood is reported as being lower in non-alcoholic individuals. The opposite is true among alcoholic individuals, in whom there is a monotonic relationship between increasing mood and higher levels of reported consumption. As in Figure 9-5, the interaction effects are highly significant.

We have just begun thinking about how we might use these consumption data as a means of case classification. One thing we have done is to see if there is a subgroup among the diagnosable subjects in whom the consumption/mood pattern is more consistent with those who do not have an alcohol diagnosis. We found that about one-third of the 22 alcoholic individuals did show such a pattern reversal, but to our surprise they actually drink more than the two-thirds who show a consistent pattern. They report heavy drinking on both low and high mood days. Although both groups of alcoholic individuals drink heavily on the weekends, those in the pattern reversal group drink more during the week. We are exploring this and other interesting patterns in these daily data.

CONCLUSION

Recently, we began to experiment with the IVR as an intervention tool for alcohol disorders and in patients with chronic pain. We are also using IVR as a tool to track progress in patients getting maintenance electroconvulsive therapy. The alcohol intervention study is the most relevant for the present context.

We are working with primary care providers to identify heavy and problem drinkers in their practices. The provider does a brief alcohol intervention as part of a regular office visit. We then enroll patients in the research project in which they call an IVR daily for 6 months to report their alcohol consumption, mood, and other variables for the previous 24 hours. Our hypothesis is that the increased vigilance will heighten and extend the impact of the brief intervention by the primary care provider. However, a by-product of this and our other IVR studies is a considerable amount of longitudinal symptomatic and behavioral data on a daily basis.

There are several potential uses of daily alcohol consumption data. It could be used to identify consumption trends, design and validate surrogate measures, identify points of intervention, monitor treatment effects, and assess time of exposure more precisely in etiological studies of such disorders as fetal alcohol syndrome. We do not know at this point how useful our IVR data will prove to be as a taxonomic tool. One concern we have is the possible restriction in the range of responses to the same questions asked day after day. This may be more of a problem for subjective reports of symptoms such as mood and stress than it is with objective behaviors such as number of alcoholic drinks. In fact, our above noted validity studies of the IVR drinking reports are reassuring. We are hopeful that a useful by-product of our current intervention research turns out to be detailed symptom information that can be used taxonomically in heavy and problem drinkers in primary care and in alcoholic individuals in specialty care settings. In fact, perhaps this tool could be used to gather useful data on those who are minimally symptomatic as well, such as the type of subjects referred to in Chapter 15. Technological advances available now, such as IVR and handheld computers, and others on the horizon, such as the transdermal alcohol sensor, which records a continuous measure of blood alcohol level (Swift 1993), provide us with new tools for ecological assessment. This in turn offers new potential for taxonomy that could help to ease the classificatory quandary we currently face between clinical convenience and scientific precision.

REFERENCES

American Psychiatric Association: Diagnostic and Statistical Manual of Mental Disorders, 4th Edition. Washington, DC, American Psychiatric Association, 1994

Epstein EE, Kahler CW, McCrady BS, et al: An empirical classification of drinking patterns among alcoholics: binge, episodic, sporadic, and steady. Addict Behav 20:23–41, 1995

Mundt JC, Searles JS, Perrine MW, et al: Cycles of alcohol dependence: frequency-domain analyses of daily drinking logs for matched alcohol dependent and non-dependent subjects. J Stud Alcohol 56:491–499, 1995

Mundt JC, Perrine MW, Searles JS: Individual differences in alcohol responsivity: physiological, psychomotor and subjective response domains. J Stud Alcohol 58:130–140, 1997

Perrine MW, Mundt JC, Searles JS, et al: Validation of daily self-reported alcohol consumption using interactive voice response (IVR) technology. J Stud Alcohol 56:487–490, 1995

Robins LN, Cotter LB, Babor T: Composite International Diagnostic Interview/ Substance Abuse Module (CIDI/SAM). St. Louis, MO, Washington University School of Medicine, 1995

Saccone NL, Kwon JM, Corbett J, et al: A genome screen of maximum number of drinks as an alcoholism phenotype. Am J Med Genet 96:632–637, 2000

Searles JS, Perrine MW, Mundt JC, et al: Self-report of drinking by touch-tone telephone: extending the limits of reliable daily contact. J Stud Alcohol 56:375–382, 1995

Searles JS, Helzer JE, Walter DE: Comparison of drinking patterns measured by daily reports and Timeline Follow Back. Psychology of Addictive Behaviors 14:277–286, 2000

Sobell LC, Sobell MB: Timeline follow-back: a technique for assessing self reported alcohol consumption, in Measuring Alcohol Consumption: Psychosocial and Biological Methods. Edited by Litten RC, Allen JP. Totowa, NJ, Humana Press, 1992, pp 41–72

Swift R: Transdermal ethanol. Addiction 88:1037–1039, 1993

10

Empirically Based Assessment and Taxonomy Across the Life Span

Thomas M. Achenbach, Ph.D.

This chapter presents an approach to psychopathology that assesses people's adaptive and maladaptive characteristics as they are reported by collaterals, observers, interviewers, and the probands themselves. The data obtained from multiple sources are then analyzed statistically to identify patterns of co-occurring characteristics that can be used to derive taxonomic constructs for psychopathology. The empirical aspects of this approach are summarized as follows:

1. Standardized procedures are used to assess problems reported for large samples of subjects.
2. Assessment data are analyzed quantitatively to detect associations among problems.
3. Syndromes are derived from identified associations among problems.
4. Scales for scoring individuals are constructed from items forming the syndromes.
5. Each scale is normed from data on large samples of subjects.
6. New cases can be evaluated via the same assessment procedures used to derive the syndromes.
7. Taxonomic constructs are formed from syndromes that are robust across samples and assessment procedures.

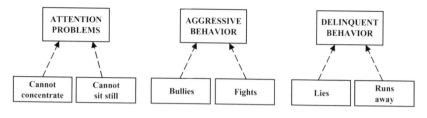

DERIVES SYNDROMES FROM STATISTICAL
ASSOCIATIONS AMONG PROBLEMS
↑
STARTS WITH DATA ON PROBLEMS

FIGURE 10-1 Empirically based "bottom up" approach to deriving syndromes from statistical associations among problems.

8. The taxonomic constructs are operationally defined in terms of scales scored from each source of data.

The empirically based approach entails multiple decisions about how to obtain data from particular sources, which sources to use, what characteristics to assess, how to analyze the data statistically, and how to use the findings. Such decisions are made in the course of long-term programmatic research that works mainly from the bottom up (Figure 10-1).

HIERARCHY OF ASSESSMENT DATA

The general strategy involves a hierarchical sequence of analyses (Figure 10-2).

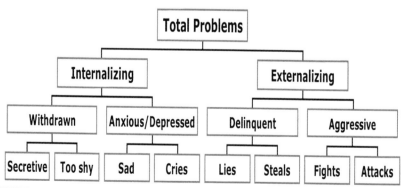

FIGURE 10-2 Hierarchy of analyses involving specific problem items, syndromes, groupings of syndromes, and total problems.

Item Scores

By working from the bottom up, my colleagues and I can organize data collected on large numbers of items in different ways. Scores on the items constitute the essential database and directly reflect informants' reports about the probands. We test the ability of each item to discriminate significantly between referred and nonreferred people.

Syndromes

To identify syndromes of co-occurring problems, we perform multivariate analyses of associations among the problem items in clinical samples. The patterns that are replicated across multiple samples according to multiple analytic criteria are used to construct syndrome scales. The word "syndrome" is used here in its generic sense to mean a set of problems that tend to occur together. An individual's score on a syndrome scale is the sum of the individual's scores on all the items of the scale.

Internalizing and Externalizing Groupings

To identify sets of syndromes that are correlated with each other, we have performed second-order factor analyses of syndromes that have yielded groupings designated as Internalizing and Externalizing. To provide a picture of whether an individual's problems are primarily Internalizing, primarily Externalizing, both, or neither, scores are computed for Internalizing and Externalizing by summing the scores on the syndromes that make up the Internalizing and Externalizing groupings.

Total Problem Score

At the highest level in the hierarchy is the total problem score, which is the sum of scores for all the problem items on the assessment instrument, regardless of whether the items are included in the syndromes. For example, some problems, such as suicidal behavior, are intrinsically important, even if they are not consistently associated with a particular syndrome. The total problem score is an exceptionally good global index of a broad spectrum of psychopathology. It is especially helpful for screening and outcome evaluations.

In sum, the diverse data that are scored at multiple levels enable clinicians and researchers to view psychopathology flexibly across levels ranging from large pools of specific problem items to smaller numbers of syndromes, broadband Internalizing and Externalizing groupings, and global total problem scores.

APPLICATIONS OF THE EMPIRICALLY BASED APPROACH

Children and Adolescents

The empirically based approach has been applied most extensively to child and adolescent psychopathology, where there has been a dearth of well-established diagnostic categories and where data must be obtained from multiple informants, such as parents, teachers, observers, and interviewers, as well as from the probands themselves (Achenbach 1995). Because children's functioning often varies from one context and interaction partner to another, correlations between different sources of data are often modest (Achenbach et al. 1987). As a consequence, comprehensive assessment requires data from multiple sources. Multiple sources of data are also needed to identify patterns of characteristics from which to derive taxonomic constructs (Figure 10-3).

After syndromes are derived, they are displayed in a profile format to facilitate assessment for both clinical and research purposes (Figure 10-4).

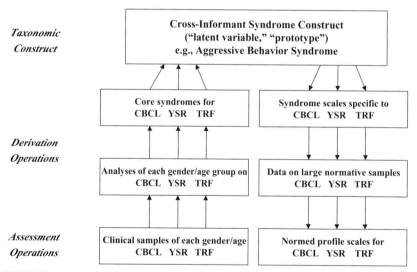

FIGURE 10-3 Derivation of cross-informant syndrome constructs from parents' ratings on the Child Behavior Checklist (CBCL), self-ratings on the Youth Self-Report (YSR), and teacher ratings on the Teacher's Report Form (TRF).

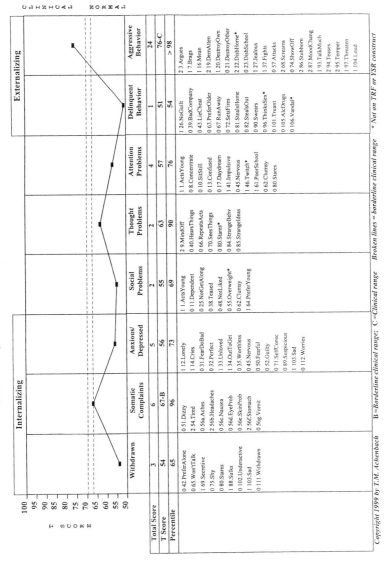

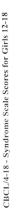

FIGURE 10-4 Windows version of syndrome profile scored from the Child Behavior Checklist (CBCL) completed by the mother of a 12-year-old girl.

Cross-Informant Comparisons

To facilitate comparisons among reports by different informants, our software provides side-by-side comparisons of scores for each item and each syndrome from up to eight informants (Figure 10-5).

To provide a quantitative index of the degree of agreement between informants, the software presents correlations between the scores obtained from each pair of informants, such as the child's mother and father, each parent with each teacher, and each adult with the child's self-reports (Figure 10-6).

Extension to Adults

The empirically based paradigm that has been extensively applied to children and adolescents is being increasingly applied to adults. We first extended this approach to subjects in our national longitudinal study when they became too old for our child and adolescent assessment instruments (Achenbach et al. 1995). We compiled large pools of items that were relevant to the transitional period from adolescence to adulthood and that could be rated by young adults about themselves and by significant others, such as parents, spouses, and friends. Because young adults may vary greatly in the pathways they follow, we included separate sets of items relevant to functioning in work, educational programs, and conjugal relationships.

From data obtained on clinical samples and a national normative sample, we derived syndromes for young adults that are displayed on profiles analogous to the child and adolescent profiles shown in Figure 10-4 (Achenbach 1997). We also constructed profiles for adaptive functioning and for substance use.

Longitudinal Findings

In our longitudinal research, we identified predictive continuities between developmentally early syndromes and young adult syndromes, as well as young adult signs of disturbance, such as suicidal behavior, substance abuse, mental health referrals, trouble with the law, and being fired from jobs (Achenbach et al. 1995, 1998). For example, Figure 10-7 shows relations between the child/adolescent Aggressive Behavior syndrome derived from parent, teacher, and self-ratings and two young adult syndromes.

One young adult syndrome is designated as Aggressive Behavior, whereas the other is designated as Intrusive. As shown in Figure 10-7, the

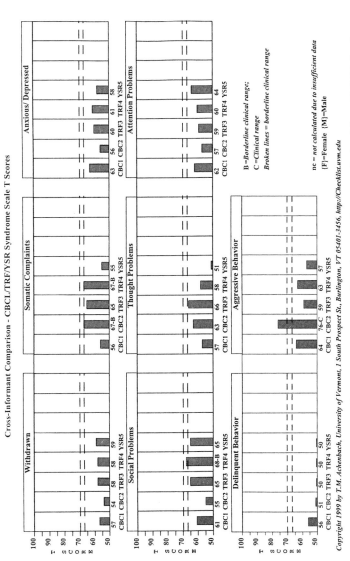

FIGURE 10-5   Windows cross-informant comparisons of syndrome scale scores obtained from Child Behavior Checklists (CBCLs), Teacher's Report Forms (TRFs), and the Youth Self-Report (YSR) for a 12-year-old girl.

Q Correlations Between Item Scores

Forms	Informants	Cross-Informant Agreement	Q Corr	Reference Group 25th %ile	Mean	75th %ile
CBC1 x CBC2	Biological Father x Biological Mother	Average	0.56	0.37	0.51	0.63
CBC1 x TRF3	Biological Father x Classroom Teacher (F)	Above average	0.39	0.07	0.19	0.30
CBC1 x TRF4	Biological Father x Classroom Teacher (F)	Above average	0.50	0.07	0.19	0.30
CBC1 x YSR5	Biological Father x Self	Above average	0.45	0.22	0.33	0.43
CBC2 x TRF3	Biological Mother x Classroom Teacher (F)	Average	0.22	0.07	0.19	0.30
CBC2 x TRF4	Biological Mother x Classroom Teacher (F)	Above average	0.36	0.07	0.19	0.30
CBC2 x YSR5	Biological Mother x Self	Average	0.38	0.22	0.33	0.43
TRF3 x TRF4	Classroom Teacher (F) x Classroom Teacher (F)	Above average	0.72	0.29	0.43	0.58
TRF3 x YSR5	Classroom Teacher (F) x Self	Above average	0.53	0.08	0.17	0.26
TRF4 x YSR5	Classroom Teacher (F) x Self	Above average	0.56	0.08	0.17	0.26

****There is no reference sample for this combination   nc = not calculated due to insufficient data

(F)=Female (M)=Male
Copyright 1999 by T.M. Achenbach, University of Vermont, 1 South Prospect St., Burlington, VT 05401-3456, http://Checklist.uvm.edu

FIGURE 10-6 Windows display of cross-informant correlations between problem item scores obtained from Child Behavior Checklists (CBCLs), Teacher's Report Forms (TRFs), and the Youth Self-Report (YSR) for a 12-year-old girl.

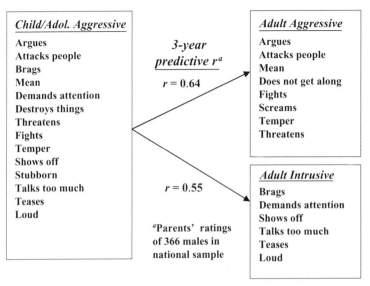

FIGURE 10-7 Predictive correlations between child/adolescent Aggressive Behavior syndrome and young adult Aggressive Behavior and Intrusive syndromes in a national sample.

adult Aggressive Behavior syndrome comprises the overtly aggressive components of the child/adolescent Aggressive Behavior syndrome, whereas the adult Intrusive syndrome comprises the socially obnoxious components of the child/adolescent syndrome. It thus appears that, during the transition to adulthood, some aggressive adolescents become less overtly aggressive while retaining their socially obnoxious behavior. Other aggressive adolescents remain overtly aggressive. This suggests that interventions may be possible to systematically reduce the more dangerous overtly aggressive behavior without the radical and perhaps impossible surgery needed to totally eliminate obnoxious behavior.

We also found an Attention Problems syndrome among young adults that was predicted by our child/adolescent Attention Problems syndrome. It is noteworthy that overactivity is no longer a part of the syndrome among young adults.

Elderly Adults

Because assessment of elderly adults often requires data from multiple sources and there is a need for a bottom-up approach to identifying patterns of adaptive and maladaptive characteristics among the elderly population, we collaborated with geriatric psychiatrists in developing an Older Adult

Behavior Checklist to be completed by family members, friends, and care-givers who know the elderly proband. We also developed a parallel Older Adult Self-Report to be completed by the probands themselves (Achenbach and Newhouse 1997).

In addition, we recently obtained data on a nationally representative sample and on multiple clinical samples from which to derive syndromes and to construct normed profiles for people who are age 60 and older. We also developed analogous self-report and other report forms for people who are ages 30 to 59, for which we obtained national normative and clinical samples (Achenbach 1998).

POTENTIAL ADVANTAGES OF THE EMPIRICALLY BASED APPROACH

The empirically based approach outlined in this chapter offers several po-tential advantages for advancing our knowledge of psychopathology for both clinical and research purposes. A fundamental advantage is that the empirically based approach starts with large pools of diverse items and then tests the ability of each item to discriminate between clinically re-ferred and nonreferred people. Items that discriminate significantly be-tween referred and nonreferred people are better candidates for assessing psychopathology than are items that do not discriminate significantly.

DSM-Oriented Options

The syndromes, Internalizing and Externalizing groupings, and total prob-lem scores that were derived from large pools of problem items scored for clinical samples were previously outlined. However, other templates also can be used to organize these pools of items. For example, many of the items have approximate counterparts among DSM criteria, and numerous stud-ies have reported significant associations between the empirically based syndromes and some DSM diagnoses (e.g., Arend et al. 1996; Edelbrock and Costello 1988; Kazdin and Heidish 1984; Morgan and Cauce 1999; Weinstein et al. 1990).

Although convergence between empirically based syndromes and DSM diagnoses is certainly of interest, the availability of scores for the prob-lem items on thousands of subjects in many samples offers some exciting new possibilities. In particular, we have had clinicians rate the degree to which each problem item on our forms is consistent with criteria for certain DSM diagnoses. Items judged to be consistent with certain DSM di-agnoses are grouped into scales. We have used data from many samples to test the discriminative power and correlates of these DSM-oriented scales.

We also have used our normative data to construct norms and cut points for the DSM-oriented scales. Clinicians and researchers can thus choose whether to have scores computed in terms of DSM-oriented scales, empirically based syndromes, or both and can compare the results obtained with DSM-oriented and empirically based scales (Achenbach and Rescorla 2001).

Cross-Cultural Research

The adaptability of our assessment instruments to diverse cultures and the diverse possibilities for analysis have facilitated translations of these instruments into 62 languages and their use in some 4,000 published studies from 50 countries (Bérubé and Achenbach 2001). Cross-cultural comparisons have been made for syndrome scores, Internalizing, Externalizing, and total problem scores from 12 cultures (Crijnen et al. 1997, 1999).

Secular Trends

Because problem levels may differ not only across cultures but also within cultures at different points in time, we compared problem scores obtained from American parents and teachers at different points in time (Figure 10–8; Achenbach and Howell 1993). Now that we have finished assessing a new national sample, we are extending our analyses of secular changes to the 23-year period from 1976 to 1999.

Genetic Research

The gender-specific norms for empirically based scales that can be scored by multiple informants over broad developmental periods offer great flexibility for many kinds of research on psychopathology. For example, behavior genetic research can benefit from the quantitative scoring of syndromes and DSM-oriented scales. This is especially helpful for research where categorical criteria for disorders yield base rates that are too low to afford adequate statistical power for testing genetic models.

Treatment Outcomes

Research on treatment outcomes can also benefit from the empirically based instruments that quantify diverse problems and adaptive characteristics prior to interventions. The same instruments can then be readministered during and after treatment to quantify changes in both the

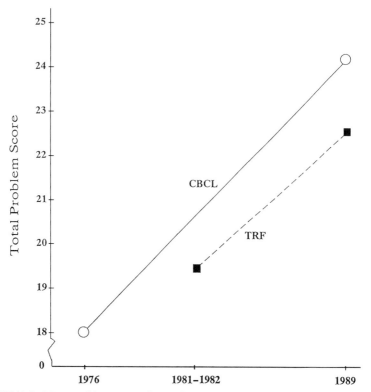

FIGURE 10-8   Mean problem scores obtained from parents on the Child Behavior Checklist (CBCL) in 1989 versus 1976 and from teachers on the Teacher's Report Form (TRF) in 1989 versus 1981–1982 (Achenbach and Howell 1993).

characteristics that were targeted for treatment and other characteristics that might be favorably or adversely affected by treatment. Gender-, age-, and instrument-specific norms and cut points enable users to determine the clinical significance of improvements according to whether patients who are initially in the clinical range reach the borderline clinical or normal range following treatment (e.g., Kendall et al. 1999).

CONCLUSION

This chapter outlines an approach to psychopathology that assesses people's adaptive and maladaptive characteristics as they are reported by collaterals, observers, interviewers, and the probands themselves. The data obtained from multiple sources are analyzed statistically to identify patterns of co-occurring characteristics on which to base taxonomic constructs for psychopathology. This approach has been applied most extensively to children and adolescents but is now being extended across the life span to elderly adults. Longitudinal studies have revealed continuities and changes from child and adolescent syndromes to adult syndromes.

The empirically based approach is compatible with other approaches, including DSM diagnoses, but it offers a variety of advantages. For example, it builds on large pools of assessment items that discriminate between clinically referred and nonreferred people, derives syndromes statistically to reflect actual patterns of co-occurring problems, identifies groupings of correlated syndromes to provide broad perspectives on patterns of psychopathology, and provides a global index of psychopathology in terms of total problem scores.

The problem items can be grouped according to alternative templates, such as those provided by DSM diagnostic criteria. The same individuals can then be scored in terms of normed scales structured according to DSM categories and to empirically based syndromes. The assessment procedures can be applied at low cost in many cultures and can quantify similarities and differences in reported problems across age, gender, cultures, and periods of time ranging up to decades. The quantification of phenotypes in terms of syndromes, DSM-oriented scales, internalizing, and externalizing also facilitates genetic research and research on the outcomes of treatment.

REFERENCES

Achenbach TM: Empirically based assessment and taxonomy: applications to clinical research. Psychol Assess 7:261–274, 1995

Achenbach TM: Manual for the Young Adult Self-Report and Young Adult Behavior Checklist. Burlington, VT, University of Vermont, Department of Psychiatry, 1997

Achenbach TM: Adult Behavior Checklist and Adult Self-Report. Burlington, VT, University of Vermont, Department of Psychiatry, 1998

Achenbach TM, Howell CT: Are American children's problems getting worse? a 13-year comparison. J Am Acad Child Adolesc Psychiatry 32:1145–1154, 1993

Achenbach TM, Newhouse P: Older Adult Behavior Checklist and Older Adult Self-Report. Burlington, VT, University of Vermont, Department of Psychiatry, 1997

Achenbach TM, Rescorla RA: Manual for the ASEBA School-Age Forms and Profiles. Burlington, VT, University of Vermont Research Center for Children, Youth, and Families, 2001

Achenbach TM, McConaughy SH, Howell CT: Child/adolescent behavioral and emotional problems: implications of cross-informant correlations for situational specificity. Psychol Bull 101:213–232, 1987

Achenbach TM, Howell CT, McConaughy SH, et al: Six-year predictors of problems in a national sample, III: transitions to young adult syndromes. J Am Acad Child Adolesc Psychiatry 34:658–669, 1995

Achenbach TM, Howell CT, McConaughy SH, et al: Six-year predictors of problems in a national sample, IV: young adult signs of disturbance. J Am Acad Child Adolesc Psychiatry 37:718–727, 1998

Arend R, Lavigne JV, Rosenbaum D, et al: Relation between taxonomic and quantitative diagnostic systems in preschool children: emphasis on disruptive disorders. J Clin Child Psychol 25:388–397, 1996

Bérubé RL, Achenbach TM: Bibliography of Published Studies Using ASEBA Instruments, 2001 Edition. Burlington, VT, University of Vermont, Department of Psychiatry, 2001

Crijnen AAM, Achenbach TM, Verhulst FC: Comparisons of problems reported by parents of children in 12 cultures: total problems, externalizing, and internalizing. J Am Acad Child Adolesc Psychiatry 36:1269–1277, 1997

Crijnen AAM, Achenbach TM, Verhulst FC: Comparisons of problems reported by parents of children in twelve cultures: the CBCL/4–18 syndrome constructs. Am J Psychiatry 156:569–574, 1999

Edelbrock C, Costello AJ: Convergence between statistically derived behavior problem syndromes and child psychiatric diagnoses. J Abnorm Child Psychol 16:219–231, 1988

Kazdin AE, Heidish IE: Convergence of clinically derived diagnoses and parent checklists among inpatient children. J Abnorm Child Psychol 12:421–435, 1984

Kendall PC, Marrs-Garcia A, Nath SR, et al: Normative comparisons for the evaluation of clinical significance. J Consult Clin Psychol 67:285–299, 1999

Morgan CJ, Cauce AM: Predicting DSM-III-R disorders from the Youth Self-Report: analysis of data from a field study. J Am Acad Child Adolesc Psychiatry 38:1237–1245, 1999

Weinstein SR, Noam GG, Grimes K, et al: Convergence of DSM-III diagnoses and self-reported symptoms in child and adolescent inpatients. J Am Acad Child Adolesc Psychiatry 29:627–634, 1990

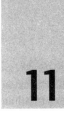

11

ADHD Comorbidity Findings From the MTA Study

New Diagnostic Subtypes and Their Optimal Treatments

Peter S. Jensen, M.D., and Members of the MTA Cooperative Group[1]

The presence of comorbid disruptive behavior disorders [conduct disorder (CD), oppositional defiant disorder (ODD)] within children diagnosed with attention-deficit hyperactivity disorder (ADHD) has been well established for almost 20 years (e.g., see Bird et al. 1990; Hinshaw 1987). Only since the 1990s has it become apparent that internalizing disorders (both anxiety and depressive disorders) also commonly co-occur with ADHD. Thus, both clinical and epidemiologic studies have consistently shown that as many as one-third of children with ADHD have co-occurring anxiety disorders (Biederman et al. 1991; Bird et al. 1990; MTA Cooperative Group 1999a; Woolston et al. 1989). This phenomenon appears

[1]Peter S. Jensen, M.D., Stephen P. Hinshaw, Ph.D., Helena C. Kraemer, Ph.D., Nilantha Lenora, B.S., Jeffrey H. Newcorn, M.D., Howard B. Abikoff, Ph.D., John S. March, M.D., L. Eugene Arnold, M.D., Dennis P. Cantwell, M.D., C. Keith Conners, Ph.D., Glen R. Elliott, M.D., Laurence L. Greenhill, M.D., Lily Hechtman, M.D., Betsy Hoza, Ph.D., William E. Pelham, Ph.D., Joanne B. Severe, M.S., James M. Swanson, Ph.D., Karen C. Wells, Ph.D., Timothy Wigal, Ph.D., Benedetto Vitiello, M.D.

This chapter represents an expanded version of a previously published article: Jensen PS, Hinshaw SP, Kraemer HC, et al.: "ADHD Comorbidity Findings From the MTA Study: Comparing Comorbid Subgroups." *Journal of the American Academy of Child and Adolescent Psychiatry* 40:147–158, 2001. Reprinted with permission of Lippincott Williams & Wilkins, Inc.

"real" and cannot be attributed *solely* to factors such as referral biases or methodologic artifacts (Angold et al. 1999).

The overlap of ADHD with both the internalizing and disruptive disorders should be of substantial interest to researchers and clinicians. For example, if it can be shown that ADHD—when comorbid with either the internalizing or disruptive disorders—is unique with respect to its clinical correlates, etiology, course, and outcome (vs. "pure" ADHD), then it may be useful to consider such comorbid states as diagnostically meaningful subtypes or even as separate disorders. Also, if various comorbid forms of ADHD are actually of qualitatively different types than "pure" ADHD, better treatment planning and clinical prediction, as well as more valid etiologic and genetic studies, should be possible.

VALIDATION OF SUBTYPES

Cantwell (1995) outlined eight domains of clinical investigation that could be used to assess the discriminate validity of possible disorder types and subtypes. These criteria, which are modified from the original Robins and Guze (1970) criteria, include 1) clinical phenomenology, 2) demographic correlates, 3) psychosocial correlates, 4) environmental family factors, 5) genetic family factors, 6) biological factors, 7) response to treatment, and (8) clinical outcomes. Applying these criteria to ADHD comorbidity studies, Jensen et al. (1997) reported that seven of the eight validational criteria supported the hypothesis that ADHD comorbid with disruptive behavior disorders (ADHD/CD-ODD) constitutes a different ADHD subtype. However, applying these same criteria to ADHD comorbid with internalizing disorders (principally anxiety), they noted somewhat weaker evidence (four of eight criteria) in support of an ADHD/Anx subtype. Since the Jensen et al. (1997) review, two additional pertinent studies have been conducted of relevance to questions concerning the usefulness and validity of the ADHD/Anx subtype. Beginning with an initial dose titration, Diamond et al. (1999) followed stimulant-treated ADHD children over 4 months to determine the impact of comorbid anxiety on ADHD children's response to medication. Unlike the preponderance of evidence from earlier studies (e.g., Buitelaar et al. 1995; DuPaul et al. 1994; Pliszka 1989, 1992; Tannock et al. 1995), Diamond and colleagues found that children with ADHD/Anx and those with ADHD/no Anx did *not* show any differential response to methylphenidate, either in terms of behavioral measures or side effects. Findings from the Multimodal Treatment Study of Children with ADHD (the MTA study), a multisite randomized clinical trial testing four treatment groups in 579 children across six sites, indicated that ADHD children with comorbid anxiety disorders have qualitatively different treatment responses than children without comorbid anxiety (MTA Cooperative Group 1999a, 1999b). Thus, among children with parent-identified anxiety disorders (33.5% of the sample), those children in the behavioral therapy condition (Beh) showed an enhanced response on outcome measures of parent-reported ADHD and internalizing symptomatology relative to nonanxious children. In addition, among anxious subjects, combined treatments (Comb) yielded greater improvements than medication management alone (MedMgt) in several outcome domains. Among nonanxious participants, however, MedMgt and Comb both outperformed Beh and the community comparison group (CC) with regard to ADHD symptoms (MTA Cooperative Group 1999b).

Findings from the MTA study (like most past studies) provide further evidence of qualitatively different treatment responses in ADHD/Anx versus ADHD/no Anx children, and may thus support the separate ADHD/Anx subtype hypothesis. In contrast, and to the surprise of the MTA investigators, the presence of comorbid CD-ODD *did not* moderate any differential treatment response to specific treatments. However, these first moderator analyses were restricted to examination of the main effects of comorbidity and did not explore possible interactions between CD-ODD and anxiety comorbidities on MTA outcomes.

Remarkably, only one study to date has examined these four potentially separate entities. In a study of 138 white males with DSM-III (American Psychiatic Association 1980)—defined ADHD, Livingston and colleagues (1990) found that boys with an internalizing disorder *and* CD-ODD differed along multiple dimensions from boys with ADHD/CD-ODD only, ADHD/Anx only, and ADHD only. In most areas of functioning, doubly comorbid boys scored worse than ADHD/CD-ODD-only and ADHD/Anx-only boys, although in at least one instance doubly comorbid boys functioned somewhat better (e.g., teacher-completed aggression ratings). Unfortunately, given the study's small sample size ($n = 138$) and its restriction to white males from one clinical setting, it could not be determined whether the differences between doubly comorbid boys and singly comorbid and ADHD-only boys were simply an additive function of the two comorbidities or whether these differences reflected unique clinical profiles.

Thus, although mounting evidence does support the possibility that comorbid ADHD/Anx and ADHD/CD-ODD individuals may have unique clinical profiles compared with noncomorbid ADHD children, firm conclusions about these comorbid patterns cannot be derived from previous research, given the relatively small sample sizes and previous studies' failures to tease apart the effects of the two comorbidities when they overlap. Furthermore, there are no previous investigations that have employed a comprehensive set of validational criteria (neither Robins and Guze [1970] nor Cantwell [1995]) to examine these potential disorder subtypes, all within the same study.

The MTA study (MTA Cooperative Group 1999a, 1999b) offers a unique opportunity to examine whether ADHD/Anx, ADHD/CD-ODD, and ADHD/Anx/CD-ODD children do indeed differ from each other and from noncomorbid ADHD children, as well as whether such findings can be replicated across multiple settings. In this report, we examine four different groups of ADHD children (ADHD/Anx, ADHD/CD-ODD, ADHD/Anx/CD-ODD, ADHD only), comparing them using the modified Cantwell validational criteria to determine if the varying forms of comorbidity convey special diagnostic, therapeutic, or outcome significance beyond the presence of ADHD alone.

METHODS

Recruitment Procedures and Sample Characteristics

MTA recruitment and screening procedures aimed to collect a carefully diagnosed, impaired sample of ADHD children with a wide range of comorbidities and demographic characteristics representative of patients seen clinically (MTA Cooperative Group 1999a). For eligibility, children (of either sex) were between ages 7.0 and 9.9 and in first through fourth grades. All met DSM-IV (American Psychiatric Association 1994) criteria for ADHD, Combined Type, using the Diagnostic Interview Schedule for Children, Parent Report, version 3.0 (DISC-P; Shaffer et al. 1996). The presence of comorbidities such as ODD, CD, internalizing disorders, or specific learning disabilities *were not* exclusions because an important aim of the MTA study was to examine their interactions with treatment outcomes.

In a four-group parallel design, 579 children were assigned randomly to 1) MedMgt, 2) Beh, 3) Comb, or 4) CC for 14 months. Demographic characteristics of the MTA participants were as follows: 80% male and 20% female; 61% white, 20% black, and 19% Hispanic, racially mixed, or other ethnic origins. Mean age at study entry was 8.2 years. Extensive information concerning subject characteristics, study treatments, and outcomes is reported elsewhere (MTA Cooperative Group 1999a, 1999b).

Assessments

The major symptom and functioning domains originally used to assess baseline characteristics and 14-month outcomes (see MTA Cooperative Group 1999a) were applied to test the Cantwell validational criteria on the various comorbidity profiles. Variables selected for the Cantwell criteria were as follows: 1) *clinical phenomenology*—inattentive, hyperactive/impulsive, and aggressive/oppositional symptoms (assessed via parent- and teacher-completed "SNAP" (an acronym for the names of the instrument's developers—Swanson, Nolan, and Pelham [see Swanson 1992]) scores; MTA Cooperative Group 1999a), verbal and performance IQ, impairment (measured via the Columbia Impairment Scale; Bird et al. 1996), internalizing symptoms [assessed via the Multidimensional Anxiety Scale for Children (MASC; March et al. 1997), the Child Depression Inventory (CDI; Kovacs and Beck 1977), and parent- and teacher-rated internalizing symptoms scales from the Social Skills Rating System (SSRS; Gresham and Elliott 1989)], and academic achievement [assessed via the Wechsler Individual Achievement Test (WIAT; Wechsler 1992)]; 2) *demographic factors*—gender, age, single-versus two-parent status, income, and family occupational status; 3) *psychosocial factors*—social skills/peer relations (assessed via parent and teacher reports using the SSRS) and levels of life stressors; 4) *family factors (both environmental and genetic)*—family stress (using the Parent Stress Index), parent-child relations [using scales from the Parent-Child Relationship questionnaire (W. Furman and T. Adler, unpublished manuscript, 1983)], parenting style based on a internally consistent and reliable factor derived from all MTA-administered parenting assessments (Wells et al. 2000), maternal depression [using the Beck Depression Inventory (BDI), Beck et al. 1961]; and 5) *biologic factors* (history of pre- and perinatal difficulties). Of note, in the original Cantwell validational scheme, *family environment* and *family genetic* factors are defined separately; here we have combined them into a single criterion because the MTA design did not provide a robust method for separating these two sources of familial effects. These five Cantwell criteria were based on data collected at the baseline assessment, allowing us to examine what Kraemer (1995) termed "epidemiologic comorbidity."

To examine the last two Cantwell criteria (*response to treatment, clinical outcomes*—also termed "clinical comorbidity" by Kraemer 1995), we constructed difference scores by subtracting 14-month endpoint scores from baseline scores of children's symptoms and functioning ratings of those variables from the *clinical phenomology, psychosocial factors*, and *family factors* domains that describe the child's functioning. In addition to these outcome measures, we also used an overall composite outcome measure (see Conners et al. 2001) to examine outcomes and response to treatment. To avoid the potentially confounding effects of the MTA treatments on more "naturalistic" outcomes, analyses of *outcomes* were limited to CC subjects only ($n = 146$), whereas *response to treatment* analyses included all subjects.

Table 11-1 details the actual proportions of subjects with each comorbidity at each of the six performance sites (A–F). These comorbidities reflect any current and past diagnoses in the last 12 months. Of note, in our first reports concerning ADHD comorbidities (MTA Cooperative Group 1999a, 1999b), simple phobia was not included in the "anxiety disorders" category, a decision initially made because of concerns that it might be normative. However, subsequent analyses have indicated that parent-reported simple phobias are in fact as likely to be validated by clinicians on re-interview as other anxiety disorders (Jensen et al. 1999). Given these findings, in this report, subjects with simple phobia were included in the "anxiety disorders" category, resulting in somewhat higher anxiety comorbidities than first reports (38.7% vs. 33.5%).

The comorbid overlap of internalizing and disruptive behaviors disorders is substantial. That is, of 294 children with CD or ODD, 42.5% ($n = 125$) had a comorbid internalizing disorder, indicating that findings attributable to CD-ODD comorbidity could instead be due to its overlap with internalizing disorders. Likewise, of 196 children with an anxiety disorder, 125 (63.7%) had concurrent CD-ODD, thereby potentially compromising conclusions one might draw about the effects of internalizing disorders on ADHD children, if such overlaps are not teased apart. Also seen in Table 11-1 are the specific proportions of subjects at each site that met criteria for ADHD only, ADHD/Anx, ADHD/CD-ODD, and ADHD/Anx/CD-ODD. To construct these groups and all subsequent comparisons, other comorbidities (e.g., enuresis, tics, mood disorders) were ignored. For the 22 cases of mood disorders in the MTA sample, all but 2 cases were comorbid with anxiety disorders. Given evidence presented by Angold et al. (1999), which showed that comorbid mood disorders in ADHD children occur principally via their association with anxiety disorders, we have named the overall category ADHD/Anx; although, in fact, this group also included two children with mood disorders who did not have a full-blown anxiety disorder.

Analytical Strategy

To determine whether ADHD children with different comorbidity profiles differed meaningfully from "pure" ADHD subjects, our analytical strategy proceeded as follows. We first coded all subjects according to the presence or absence of the two comorbidity forms (i.e., presence or absence of anxiety comorbidity ["Anx"] and CD-ODD comorbidity ["CD-ODD"]). Then, to examine the potential distinctions between the singly comorbid groups (e.g., ADHD/Anx) and the doubly comorbid group (ADHD/Anx/CD-ODD), it was necessary to determine whether the effects of each comorbidity applied

TABLE 11-1 MTA subjects' baseline comorbidity characteristics by site

Disorder frequency (%) (with impairment)*	Total sample $n = 579$ (%)	Per site** (%)					
		A $n = 95$	B $n = 96$	C $n = 96$	D $n = 98$	E $n = 96$	F $n = 98$
Anxiety disorders	38.7	40.0	44.8	39.6	38.7	40.6	28.6
Conduct disorder (CD)	14.4	16.8	7.4	13.5	19.4	15.6	13.3
Oppositional defiant disorder (ODD)	42.4	42.5	47.8	44.9	40.4	30.5	48.4
Affective disorder	6.3	9.7	7.2	3.3	10.4	4.2	1.1
Tic disorders	11.6	15.1	10.0	13.3	12.4	7.2	11.2
Other (i.e., bulimia, enuresis)	0.4	0	2.2	0	0	0	0
Percent with ADHD-only	31.8	31.6	30.2	32.3	26.5	34.4	35.7
Percent with ADHD/Anx	14.0	12.6	17.7	12.5	17.3	19.8	4.1
Percent with ADHD/CD-ODD	29.5	28.4	25.0	28.1	34.7	25.0	35.7
Percent with ADHD/Anx/CD-ODD	24.7	27.4	27.1	27.1	21.4	20.8	24.5

Note. *Only disorders with impairment were counted; **Chi square values were not significant by either site or treatment group.

equally across its single and doubly comorbid forms (termed a "main effect" of that comorbidity), or whether any interaction effects (Anx × CD-ODD) existed. These issues were explored on all Cantwell criteria via multivariate analyses, examining the extent to which Anx, CD-ODD, and Anx × CD-ODD effects could be found for specific indicators. If these analyses demonstrate multiple Anx × CD-ODD interactions, or indicate that when Anx and CD-ODD effects are found, they usually occur with different variables, such findings would provide evidence for the need to discriminate among the three potential comorbid subgroups versus "pure" ADHD-only subjects.

To further examine the *response to treatment* criterion, we constructed unique codes for each MTA treatment group assignment. Then, using these codes in multivariate analyses of the difference scores described earlier, along with codes for the four comorbidity subtypes, we examined all interactions between comorbidity subtype and MTA treatment group status in the final model. Finding interactions between a given MTA treatment and any comorbidity group would have important implications for treatment planning and could enhance clinicians' abilities to match patients to specific treatments.

Finally, to determine clinical significance of all findings, effect sizes were computed to examine the impact of comorbidity subtypes on baseline characteristics, outcomes, and response to treatment.

Given our concern that too stringent methods might result in failure to identify modest to moderate effects within relatively small comorbidity groups stratified across six sites and four treatment conditions, P values were set at a modest $P < 0.05$ and no corrections for multiple tests were performed. After statistical consultation, we reasoned that this was a defensible strategy because these are exploratory analyses and the interpretation of results should not rest on any single statistical analysis per se. Thus, readers are encouraged to exercise caution in the interpretation of findings. For all analyses, because previous analyses (MTA Cooperative Group 1999b) demonstrated that neither gender nor ethnicity significantly affected results, these two variables were not included as covariates. In contrast, because important differences in baseline characteristics have been found across sites, site status was entered as a covariate for all analyses.

RESULTS

Results are presented in the following order: 1) head-to-head comparisons of the two singly comorbid subtypes [to determine whether the specific *kind* of comorbidity (Anx or CD-ODD) makes a difference]; 2) examination of CD-ODD and Anx main, additive, and/or interaction effects by applying Cantwell criteria across baseline characteristics and outcomes;

3) examination of possible differential benefits of specific treatments on specific comorbid groups' outcomes; and 4) examination of effect sizes.

Do ADHD/Anx and ADHD/CD-ODD Subjects Differ?

Table 11-2 presents the baseline means from each of the four groups constructed by comorbidity profiles. No analyses are presented for any baseline variables that simply reflect how the groups were formed (e.g., parent/teacher reports of aggression/oppositionality and internalizing symptoms). The comparisons of the two nonoverlapping ADHD comorbidity profiles (ADHD/Anx, ADHD/CD-ODD) can be seen in the second and third columns from the left in Table 11-2 (baseline characteristics, Cantwell criteria 1–5). Significant differences between these two groups are indicated by underlining and bold type. Inspection of these columns indicates that these two singly comorbid groups differed in 11 instances on baseline characteristics (Table 11-2).

Due to space considerations, analyses of the *outcomes* criterion are not presented here. Nonetheless, findings from ADHD/Anx versus ADHD/CD-ODD outcome comparisons overlapped substantially with, and were consistent with, the analogous differences noted between these two comorbid groups at baseline for five variables (parent-rated subscale and total scores on the SNAP, overall impairment, WIAT math, and Conners' composite scores). In addition, for three additional variables—all teacher-completed (SNAP inattention, total SNAP scores, and SSRS social skills)—significant differences were found between ADHD/Anx and ADHD/CD-ODD subjects' outcomes (tabled data available on request from the first author by email [pj131@columbia.edu]).

The differences between these two comorbid groups cross many areas of functioning, including domains where ADHD/CD-ODD subjects were more impaired (e.g., baseline hyperactive-impulsive symptoms, overall impairment, parent-child relations, and the composite index), as well as other quite different areas of functioning where ADHD/Anx subjects were more impaired (e.g., baseline academic performance scores, likelihood of a learning disability diagnosis, less improvement in teacher-rated inattention by 14 months, and less improvement in the composite index).

Are the Two Forms of Comorbidity Simply "Additive?"

Turning to the multivariate analyses to explore additive and interactive effects of the two forms of comorbidity, columns 2 through 4 from the right in Table 11-2 indicate significant main (Anx, CD-ODD) and interactive

TABLE 11-2 Validation criteria by comorbidity subtype—mean scores and effect sizes

| | Subtype mean scores | | | | Effect sizes | | | |
Variable	ADHD*	+ Anx	+ CD-ODD	+ Dual	Anx*	CD*	CD × Anx*	Pooled SD
n's =	184	81	171	143				
Clinical Phenomenology (baseline)								
Inattentive (T)	2.27	2.28	2.21	2.16	-.02	.09	.09	(F = 1.42, P < .20; 8,560) .652
Inattentive (P)	1.92	2.10	2.12	2.08	-.29	-.32	.35	(F = 2.74, P < .006; 8,563) .627
Hyperactive/Impulsive (T)	2.00	1.87	2.04	2.01	.17	-.05	-.13	(F = 1.82, P < .07; 8,563) .765
Hyperactive/Impulsive (P)	1.72	_1.87_	_2.04_	2.05	-.20	-.43[3]	.19	(F = 4.94, P < .005; 8,565) .751
Total SNAP (T)	1.76	1.75	1.85	1.85	.02	-.18[1]	.02	(F = 2.76, P < .005; 8,547) .512
Total SNAP (P)	1.46	_1.59_	_1.80_	1.86	-.26[1]	-.69[3]	.14	(F = 10.5, P < .001; 8,551) .494
CDI (Child)	0.39	0.42	0.41	0.37	-.10	-.06	.23	(F = 1.72, P < .09; 8,567) .311
MASC (Child)	2.52	2.57	2.46	2.52	-.09	.11	-.02	(F = 1.32, P < .23; 8,536) .532
Columbia Impairment Scale (P)	18.0	_21.0_	_23.8_	27.5	-.38[3]	-.74[3]	-.09	(F = 17.4, P < .001; 8,422) 7.83
Child Needs Services (P)	2.87	3.09	3.33	3.49	-.26[1]	-.54[3]	.07	(F = 5.10, P < .001; 8,422) .853
LD Diagnosis (yes/no) (proportion)	0.16	_0.22_	_0.13_	0.13	-.17[3]	.08	.17	(F = 1.16, P < .33; 8,570) .361
IQ Verbal	101	100	101	101	-.07	.00	-.07	(F = 1.89, P < 0.06; 8,564) 14.8
Performance	102	101	102	100	-.06	.00	.06	(F = 2.47, P < .012; 8,564) 15.6
WIAT Math	99.2	_94.5_	_99.1_	96.7	-.34[2]	-.01	.17	(F = 3.38, P < .001; 8,570) 13.8
WIAT Spelling	95.8	_91.0_	_94.4_	93.1	-.34[1]	-.10	.25	(F = 2.04, P < .04; 8,570) 14.0
WIAT Reading	96.9	93.5	96.4	94.9	-.24[2]	-.04	.13	(F = 1.43, P < .19; 8,570) 14.2
Overall composite score	0.94	_2.64_	_6.96_	8.68	-.21[2]	-.76[3]	-.00	(F = 17.1, P < .001; 8,570) 7.94
Demographic Factors (baseline)								
Gender (proportion male)	.80	.79	.81	.81	-.03	.03	.03	(F = 1.44, P < .18; 8,570) .40
Age (in years)	7.8	_7.5_	_7.8_	7.9	-.37[2]	.00	.50[1]	(F = 2.27, P < .03; 8,570) .808
Minority (yes/no) (proportion)	.34	.44	.40	.41	-.20	-.12	.18	(F = 13.7, P < .001; 8,568) .489
Two parents in home (proportion)	.75[(1.7)]	.56[(1.5)]	.70[(1.7)]	.59[(1.5)]	-.35[2]	.00	.00	(F = 3.79, P < .001; 8,570) .567
Income (proportion on welfare status)	.12	.21	.20	.27	-.23[1]	-.20	.10	(F = 7.07, P < .001; 8,570) .393

Psychosocial Factors (baseline)

	ADHD	+Anx	+CD-ODD	+Dual	Anx	CD	Anx × CD	F	ES
Social skills/Peer relations									
SSRS (T)	0.86	0.84	0.80	0.80	−.07	−.22	.07	[F = 2.15, P < .03; 8,531]	.278
SSRS (P)	1.11	1.06	0.98	0.94	−.21[1]	−.55[3]	.04	[F = 8.01, P < .001; 8,514]	.235
# of life stressors (all neg. events)***	2.0	2.3	2.5	3.1	−.12	−.21[2]	−.12	[F = 2.84, P < .004; 8,560]	2.42
# of life stressors (confounded)	1.2	1.4	1.6	2.0	−0.11	−0.21[2]	−0.11	[F = 3.37, P < .001; 8,560]	1.90
Family factors (environmental and genetic, baseline)									
Wells Parenting Index (P)	0.15	**0.68**	**−0.48**	0.03	**.29[2]**	**−.34[3]**	−.01	[F = 3.96, P < .001; 8,575]	1.84
Parenting Stress Index (P)	3.64	3.49	3.37	3.20	**−.28[3]**	**−.50[3]**	.04	[F = 8.78, P < .001; 8,515]	.535
Parent-Child (Power Assertion) (P)	2.58	2.63	**2.83**	2.82	−.09	**−.46[3]**	.09	[F = 4.18, P < .001; 8,552]	.542
Parent-Child (Positive Affection) (P)	3.60	3.64	**3.46**	3.57	.08	**−.28[1]**	.14	[F = 1.61, P < .119; 8,552]	.494
Maternal Depression (BDI) (P)	.27	.35	.29	.39	**−.28[3]**	−.07	−.07	[F = 3.22, P < .001; 8,518]	.291
Biologic factors									
# of prenatal problems	1.5	1.4	1.4	1.2	.07	.07	.07	[F = 1.25, P < .27; 8,570]	1.37
# of perinatal problems	0.5	0.6	0.5	0.7	**−.13[1]**	.00	−.13	[F = 2.23, P < 0.03; 8,570]	.77
Total pre-perinatal problems	1.9	2.0	1.9	1.9	−.06	.00	.06	[F = 0.56, P < 0.81; 8,570]	1.72
Mat. postpartum depressive sx.	2.0	2.2	1.9	2.1	−.18	.09	.00	[F = 1.39, P < .20; 8,530]	1.11

Note. For scale scores, higher scores and positive values indicate improvement/better functioning; negative scores indicate deterioration. [1]$P \leq .05$; [2]$P \leq .01$; [3]$P < .001$.

*ADHD, +Anx, +CD-ODD, and +Dual represent the 4 comorbidity groups, classified based on presence or absence of each comorbidity. Anx, CD: represent the dummy codes for presence/absence of each comorbidity coded and entered in multivariate analyses. Significant main effects and interactions (Anx × CD) for comorbidity are denoted in the respective columns by bolding the respective effect sizes and use of footnote[1,2,3] to indicate level of statistical significance.

**Key to Abbreviations: T = teacher; P = parent; ES = effect size; CDI = Child Depression Inventory; MASC = Multidimensional Anxiety Scale for Children; LD = Learning disability; WIAT = Wechsler Individual Achievement Test; SSRS = Social Skills Rating Scale; BDI = Beck Depression Inventory.

***Stress scores were computed based first by summing only those events that were not potentially a result of subjects' or families, own functioning ("unconfounded"), then by summing only those events that may in fact result from families' functioning e.g., divorce or parental separation ("confounded") (See Jensen et al. 1993).

(Anx × CD-ODD) effects. Significant effects are bolded and marked with su-perscripts 1, 2, or 3 to denote levels of significance. There were 22 variables for which there were significant effects of comorbidity on baseline charac-teristics, and 7 additional instances of effects of comorbidity on outcomes (not shown here, but available on request). Of note, across these variables, only 7 instances of additive effects of comorbidity were found (character-ized by significant effects being noted in columns 6 and 7—parent total SNAP scores, overall impairment, need for services, parent-rated social skills, the Parenting Stress Index, the Wells parenting factor, and the com-posite index). Note that none of the measures, except the parent total SNAP scores, attempt to measure psychopathology directly; rather, they are gen-eral indices of the overall impact of psychopathology on impairment, need for services, and families. These findings indicate that, although the two different forms of comorbidity/psychopathology are not additive per se, their combined impact on external factors such as overall impairment, family burden, and services use may be.

Apart from the seven variables where additive effects were found, find-ings from Table 11-2 and our *outcome* criterion analyses revealed that Anx comorbidity exerted main effects on either baseline or outcome variables in 12 instances, whereas CD-ODD exerted effects on 9 other variables. Thus, the most common main effects of Anx and CD-ODD comorbidities were noted on different variables, suggesting quite different symptom profiles of subjects, depending on their particular comorbidity subtype.

Do Comorbid Subtypes Differ in Response to Specific Treatments?

Table 11-3 presents findings concerning the *response to treatment* criterion among all three MTA-delivered interventions (vs. CC) examined via the multivariate analyses. Turning first to the issue of unique effects of possi-ble subtypes, such patterns are revealed by letters B (Beh), M (MedMgt), and C (Comb) in the columns denoting the comorbidity subtypes. All comor-bidity group effects are presented vis-à-vis comparisons to the ADHD-only group. Likewise, treatment effects are presented with reference to the CC group. Of note in the table are the commonly found, differentially beneficial effects of Beh interventions for the ADHD/Anx group. These interactions are indicative of treatment effects *over and above the main effects* of all treatments for the entire sample (irrespective of comorbidity), beyond Beh treatment benefits for the entire sample, and even distinct from the impact of Comb and Med treatments on the ADHD/Anx subgroup itself.

The second finding revealed in Table 11-3 is that dually comorbid sub-jects also evidence a substantial benefit to specific treatments, sometimes

TABLE 11-3 Response to treatment by comorbidity subtypes (difference scores = baseline minus 14 months)

	ADHD	+Anx	+CD-ODD	+Dual	Main effects of comorbid group on outcomes	Statistics
$n =$	184	81	171	143		
Inattentive (T)	.90	.78 B, M	.83	.91		[F = 1.47, P < .09; 20,557]
Inattentive (P)	.71	.77 B	.81	.78 B	ADHD/Anx	[F = 3.44, P < .001; 20,555]
Hyp/Impulsive (T)	.98	.85	.93	.99		[F = 1.64, P < .04; 20,557]
Hyp/Impulsive (P)	.70	.79 B	.86	.81 C		[F = 4.01, P < .001; 20,555]
Opp. Aggressive (T)	.49	.42 B	.54	.62		[F = 1.68, P < .03; 20,557]
Opp. Aggressive (P)	.29	.31	.55	.58	ADHD/Anx/CD-ODD	[F = 3.08, P < .001; 20,555]
Total SNAP Sx (T)	.78	.64 B, M	.75	.85		[F = 2.22, P < .002; 20,557]
Total SNAP Sx (P)	.56	.59 B	.70	.70 B	ADHD/Anx/CD-ODD	[F = 4.45, P < .001; 20,555]
Aggression (P)	.05	.05	.09	.11	ADHD/CD-ODD	[F = 1.59, P < .05; 20,558]
Internalizing Sx (T)	.12	.24 M	.15	.07	ADHD/Anx	[F = 1.55, P < .06; 20,524]
Internalizing Sx (P)	.15	.14 B	.22	.32 B	ADHD/Anx/CD-ODD	[F = 3.34, P < .001; 20,547]
MASC (Child)	.23	.25	.25	.16		[F = 1.17, P < .27; 20,524]
CDI (Child)	.15	.14	.14	.11		[F = 1.40, P < .12; 20,555]
Columbia Imp. Scale	5.8	5.4 B	7.6	9.7	ADHD/Anx/CD-ODD	[F = 4.23, P < .001; 20,470]
Needs Services (P)	.76	.95	.67	.92		[F = 2.92, P < .001; 20,558]
Social skills (T)	.23	.24 B	.25	.30		[F = 1.68, P < .03; 20,519]
Social skills (P)	.14	.06	.16	.17		[F = 1.55, P < .05; 20,548]
Overall composite	7.5	8.5 B	9.1	8.6 B	ADHD/Anx,	[F = 4.41, P < .001; 20,558]
P-C Power Assertion	.22	.20	.32	.31	ADHD/Anx/CD-ODD	[F = 1.50, P < .08; 20,544]
P-C Pos. Affection	.01	.07	.04	.05		[F = 0.70, P < .83; 20,544]
WIAT Math	2.5	3.7 B	1.0 B,M	2.5		[F = 1.55, P < .06; 20,558]
WIAT Spelling	0.7	2.7 B,C	1.0	1.0	ADHD/Anx	[F = 0.94, P < .53; 20,558]
WIAT Reading	1.4	1.2	1.4	1.2		[F = 1.48, P < .08; 20,558]
LD @14 mo. (proportion)	.10	.16	.08	.16		[F = 1.28, P < .19; 20,558]
ADHD at 14 mo.	.42	.57	.50	.55		[F = 3.63, P < .001; 20,558]

Note. **B, M, C:** Bolded figures indicate that the MTA treatment type (B = Beh, M = MedMgt, C = Comb) exerted different effects on the particular comorbidity group in that column compared to the overall effects of that same treatment for all subjects irrespective of comorbidity profile.

Comb, sometimes Beh, whereas ADHD/CD-ODD subjects rarely showed a differential response to any of the treatments compared with ADHD-only subjects.

The right column of Table 11-3 indicates whether there were any main effects of comorbidity group subtype on outcomes. Of note, seven of these eight instances were of subjects with comorbid anxiety (ADHD/Anx or ADHD/Anx/CD-ODD subtypes), with inspection of means revealing that these two groups generally showed the greatest response to treatments (tables available from the authors on request), regardless of treatment type.

How Large and Clinically Meaningful Are Comorbidity Subtype Effects?

The size and statistical significance of comorbidity effects on baseline characteristics (Table 11-2) can be seen in the right-sided column of the table. Review of Table 11-2 suggests that the effects of CD-ODD comorbidity are generally more pronounced than Anx effects on baseline characteristics and are generally associated with greater levels of symptoms (e.g., hyperactive-impulsive symptoms), lower levels of functioning (teacher-rated social skills), and overall impairment. Important exceptions were noted in academic functioning, where ADHD/Anx subjects evidenced sizeable effects with lower functioning levels. Further review of this table also indicates that in almost all instances of additive effects of the two comorbidities (parent total SNAP scores, impairment, need for services, teacher-rated social skills, and the composite index), effects exerted by CD-ODD were twofold or more larger than those conveyed by Anx. Analyses of effect sizes of the *outcomes* criterion revealed few instances of comorbidity effects on outcomes independent of MTA treatments. Important exceptions were the relative lack of improvement over time in teacher-reported inattention and the overall composite index among ADHD/Anx and ADHD/Anx/CD-ODD subjects (table available on request).

Effect sizes based on comorbidity profiles on the *treatment response* criterion are much more complex because any given variable could have 12 different effect sizes (3 MTA treatments × 4 comorbidity profiles). Therefore, effect sizes for selected variables where *comorbidity × treatment* interactions were noted in Table 11-3 are presented in graphic form in Figure 11-1. Review of Figure 11-1 indicates that ADHD/Anx subjects are particularly responsive to Beh, compared with subjects in other comorbidity groups, which rarely did as well (i.e., ES > 0.4) with Beh alone. Figure 11-1 also indicates that ADHD/Anx/CD-ODD subjects were preferentially responsive to Comb interventions, as indicated by a robust

SNAP Inattention (parent)

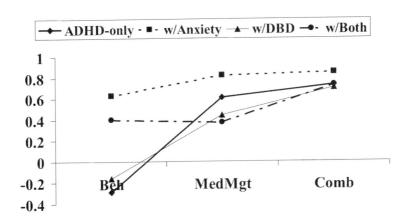

SNAP Inattention (teacher)

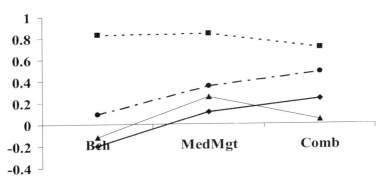

FIGURE 11-1   Effect sizes of MTA treatment by comorbidity group—selected 14-month outcomes. See Table 11-3 for *F* statistics and *P* values.

response (ES = 0.92) to Comb and much lower ES for Beh (0.53) and MedMgt (0.28) in the overall composite rating. By and large, the effect sizes of ADHD-only and ADHD/CD-ODD subjects were generally lower than those for ADHD/Anx and ADHD/Anx/CD-ODD subjects. For ADHD-only and ADHD/CD-ODD subjects, Beh alone interventions never appeared beneficial.

SNAP Total (parent)

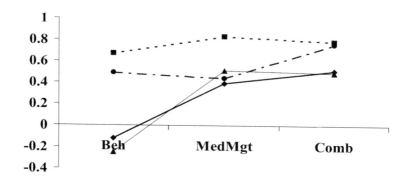

SNAP Total (teacher)

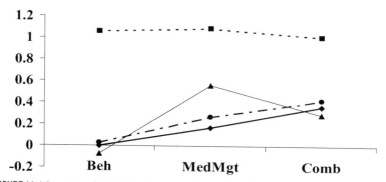

FIGURE 11-1 *(continued)*   Effect sizes of MTA treatment by comorbidity group—selected 14-month outcomes. See Table 11-3 for F statistics and P values.

DISCUSSION

Our findings suggest that ADHD children with and without CD-ODD and Anx differed on many baseline characteristics, outcomes, and response to treatment. Although CD-ODD comorbidity commonly exerted fairly

Overall Impairment

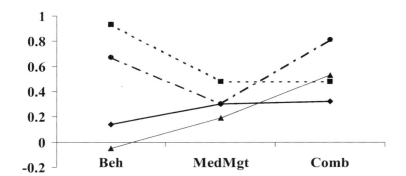

Composite Index

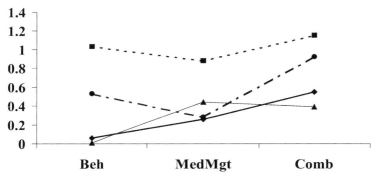

FIGURE 11-1 *(continued)*   Effect sizes of MTA treatment by comorbidity group—selected 14-month outcomes. See Table 11-3 for *F* statistics and *P* values.

powerful main effects on baseline characteristics, it rarely interacted with treatment response or outcomes. In contrast, Anx conditions exerted somewhat less robust effects on baseline characteristics but frequently interacted with response to specific treatments. Concerning our subtype hypothesis, although both Anx and CD-ODD frequently exerted straightforward main effects, their effects did not usually operate on the same variables. Thus, such effects were found in only six instances of all variables examined, and these variables pertained more to the *impact of psychopathology* than psychopathology per se. Taken together, our findings—consistent differences between ADHD/Anx and ADHD/CD-ODD groups, rarely found additive effects, the impact of CD-ODD and Anx on different variables, and the differential impact of specific treatments on the four comorbidity types, with some but not all treatments yielding effects of sizeable magnitude—indicate that the overall clinical profiles of the comorbidity types are sufficiently distinct to support the need to discriminate among the comorbid subgroups.

Consistent with our first report of anxiety as a moderating variable on outcomes (MTA Cooperative Group 1999b), we found substantial, recurring indications of Anx comorbidity (either alone or in interaction with CD-ODD) moderating responses to treatment. In addition, however, this analysis, going well beyond our earlier report, suggests that anxiety may interact with treatment outcomes across many more variables than first described, more readily detectable here with Anx × CD-ODD interactions included in the analytic model.

It is of interest to note that Anx exerted relatively modest effects on baseline characteristics and outcomes yet exerted persistent, sometimes sizeable effects on *response to treatment* findings. Reasons for this finding are unclear but could be due to the simple fact that behavioral interventions are selectively effective for ADHD children with parent-defined anxiety and that these children are qualitatively different in terms of etiologic processes and developmental trajectories. The possibility of qualitative differences in these children is further supported by the findings of WIAT score differences seen in these subjects at baseline, increased frequency of baseline demographic factors that might be expected to be linked to anxiety (e.g., more single parent homes, increased welfare status), as well as evidence from other reports that such children may have different physiologic reactions to methylphenidate (Urman et al. 1995).

As a general rule, Anx status appeared to confer certain benefits on ADHD children, regardless of the presence of CD-ODD. Thus, inspection of Table 11-2 and our *outcomes* criterion analyses (available on request) indicates that most (40 of 58) CD-ODD × Anx interaction effects were positive (although rarely significant); that is, they exerted ameliorating effects on concurrent CD-ODD (i.e., ADHD/Anx/CD-ODD vs. ADHD/CD-ODD subjects). Furthermore, Figure 11-1 indicates that children with Anx tended to be more treatment responsive than those with ADHD/CD-ODD and even ADHD-only subjects, both in terms of absolute effect sizes and in terms of their relatively robust response to all treatment modalities. The ADHD/Anx group in particular responded to almost any of the three treatments, with the single exception of academic performance, in which possible adverse effects of medication management were noted in the ADHD/Anx group. This is of some interest given historical reports of adverse effects of medication treatments on learning. In contrast, in a number of important instances, ADHD/Anx/CD-ODD subjects appeared to derive substantially greater benefits from Comb interventions compared with all other treatments, thus providing some justification of their separate classification from ADHD/Anx subjects.

ADHD-only and ADHD/CD-ODD subjects usually responded only to interventions that included medication. Although ADHD-only and ADHD/CD-ODD subjects appeared quite similar in terms of degree of clinical change in response to treatment and outcomes, the sizable baseline differences in severity between these two groups indicate a more problematic prognosis for the ADHD/CD group. In fact, additional analyses of outcomes and response to treatment based solely on absolute levels of 14-month symptoms (rather than difference scores) revealed that these two groups continued to show substantial differences at endpoint on a number of critical variables, such as parent-reported aggression, need for services, impairment, social skills, and parent-child relations, and the overall composite index (tables available from the authors on request). These persistent differences in prognosis may justify the separate classification of these two profiles.

Limitations

In consideration of our findings, a number of caveats must be carefully weighed. First, ours was a referred sample, so any inferences that these findings are applicable to ADHD comorbidity patterns in the general community are not warranted. In addition, our analyses of the *outcomes* criterion "independent of treatment" (i.e., with CC subjects only) must be viewed with caution because most CC subjects did indeed obtain some form of treatment, and our preliminary findings suggest that those seeking treatment benefited slightly more than those who did not seek care (MTA Cooperative Group 1999a, 1999b).

Another word of caution is warranted concerning those analyses, suggesting differential response to treatments as a function of comorbidity, particularly anxiety. As noted elsewhere, little overlap is found between parent- and child-identified anxiety syndromes (e.g., Jensen et al. 1999). This issue is of consequence because our additional analyses (March et al. 2000) of the moderator effects of anxiety on MTA outcomes indicate that, in contrast to parent-reported anxiety comorbidity, child-reported anxiety syndromes exert little if any moderating effects on MTA outcomes. Thus, it remains unclear whether the moderating effects of anxiety reported here apply to anxiety disorders per se or to some broader construct of parent-identified behavioral and affective dysregulation. Relatedly, we found substantially lower rates of affective disorder in the MTA sample than have been reported in other clinical studies (e.g., Biederman et al. 1991), raising concerns about the possibility of substantial underdiagnosis of these conditions, as well as any definitive conclusions about the impact of single versus multiple comorbidities on putative ADHD subtypes.

We note that our decision to combine CD and ODD cases into a single disruptive disorder category is not without controversy. On the one hand, evidence from clinical studies suggests that most ADHD children with comorbid CD also often meet criteria for ODD, which has in fact usually preceded CD onset by several years (e.g., Biederman et al. 1996). On the other hand, a number of population-based studies have suggested that ODD and CD, while intercorrelated 0.70 to 0.76, may nonetheless constitute somewhat separate dimensions of psychopathology (Quay 1999). Our decision to combine these two disorders reflects in part the substantial (but incomplete) overlap between the two disorders, as well the lack of power to examine CD as a separate disorder, given our sample sizes.

A final note of caution concerns the use of clinical samples to explore comorbidity. As noted by Angold et al. (1999), clinical samples can be burdened by methodological artifacts, potentially leading to incorrect estimates of comorbidity rates and even mistaken etiologic inferences. Nonetheless, clinical studies of comorbidity can be useful to the extent that the conclusions from such studies are intended to apply only to other clinical samples. In this regard, the MTA's inclusion and exclusion criteria, such as admitting only children with *ADHD Combined Type* and excluding children with psychosis, Tourette's syndrome, or concurrently being treated with antipsychotic medications, demarcate some of the possible limitations concerning inferences that might be drawn to more heterogeneous clinical samples.

Despite the possible referral biases that may have characterized our clinical sample, we note that our findings were obtained from multiple socioeconomic, gender, and ethnic groups across six different performance sites, whereas site factors were controlled, suggesting that these findings may be applicable to other clinically selected groups of ADHD children, combined subtype. Ours is the first empirical application of the Robins and Guze/Cantwell criteria to these comorbidity subtypes. Follow-up studies might usefully employ epidemiological sampling designs to determine the extent to which findings are applicable to unselected/nonreferred populations. Unfortunately, such studies often prove difficult to mount, given the potential sample sizes needed to examine these comorbidity patterns with sufficient power, as well as other challenges common to such studies, such as less comprehensive assessment batteries. Regardless, additional research to further discriminate these subtypes may be warranted, with future studies examining potential differentiating etiologic, neuropsychological, environmental, and genetic factors.

Clinical Implications

Our findings may have considerable implications for future research and treatment studies, as well as for the clinical process of matching of patients to treatments. As constructed, our comorbidity groups appear to differ in a number of areas, including several notable baseline characteristics, response to treatment, and outcomes. ADHD children with parent-defined anxiety disorders, particularly those with no accompanying CD-ODD, may have a number of unique characteristics, most notably seen in WIAT performance scores at baseline (also reported by Livingston et al. 1990) and at 14 months. In addition, this group evinces a clinical profile that is not a simple function of how it was originally formed (persistent ADHD, teacher-reported inattention at 14 months), and perhaps most important, in its differential response to treatment. Although the discriminating responses to treatments (especially the behavioral components of Beh and Comb) were frequently shared between the ADHD/Anx and ADHD/Anx/CD groups (suggesting a main effect of Anx status), additional interactions with treatment response were found by separating Anx children into the ADHD/Anx and ADHD/Anx/CD groups, compared with our original report (MTA Cooperative Group 1999b).

A simple "rule of thumb" that summarizes these findings suggests that if a child presents with an ADHD/Anx profile, *all* interventions are likely to be effective. If a child presents with ADHD only or ADHD/CD-ODD, treatments with medication appear especially indicated, and Beh alone strategies may be contraindicated. Finally, if a child presents with ADHD/Anx/CD-ODD, Comb interventions may offer substantial advantages over other treatments, particularly in overall impairment and functioning outcomes.

Our findings suggest that more precise matching of patients to treatment using patients' comorbidity profiles may mitigate initial clinical uncertainty, reduce the number of therapeutic trials until a workable treatment is found, and yield larger treatment gains for specific patients. Future pathophysiologic and genetic studies may benefit by these discriminations to the extent that these clinical profiles reflect different etiologic and developmental processes. Our findings, although exploratory and subject to the limitations of clinical sampling biases, constitute the first comprehensive application of the Robins and Guze/Cantwell criteria to several potential ADHD subtypes across multiple settings. Pending additional confirmatory studies, as well as further validational studies of parent-versus child-reported anxiety disorders, developers of DSM-V should consider the development of three new ADHD subtypes: ADHD/Anx (no CD-ODD), ADHD/CD-ODD (no Anx), and ADHD/Anx/CD-ODD.

Acknowledgments. The MTA is a cooperative treatment study performed by six independent research teams in collaboration with the staff of the Division of Services and Intervention Research of the National Institute of Mental Health (NIMH), Rockville, Maryland, and the Office of Special Education Programs (OSEP) of the U.S. Department of Education (DOE). The NIMH Principal Collaborators are Peter S. Jensen, M.D., L. Eugene Arnold, M.Ed., M.D., John E. Richters, Ph.D., Joanne B. Severe, M.S., Donald Vereen, M.D., and Benedetto Vitiello, M.D. Principal Investigators and Coinvestigators from the six sites are as follows: University of California at Berkeley/San Francisco (UO1 MH50461): Stephen P. Hinshaw, Ph.D., Glen R. Elliott, M.D., Ph.D.; Duke University (UO1 MH50447): C. Keith Conners, Ph.D., Karen C. Wells, Ph.D., John S. March, M.D., M.P.H.; University of California at Irvine/Los Angeles (UO1 MH50440): James M. Swanson, Ph.D., Dennis P. Cantwell, M.D., Timothy Wigal, Ph.D.; Long Island Jewish Medical Center/Montreal Children's Hospital (UO1 MH50453): Howard B. Abikoff, Ph.D., Lily Hechtman, M.D.; New York State Psychiatric Institute/Columbia University/Mount Sinai Medical Center (UO1 MH50454): Laurence L. Greenhill, M.D., Jeffrey H. Newcorn, M.D.; University of Pittsburgh (UO1 MH50467): William E. Pelham, Ph.D., Betsy Hoza, Ph.D. Helena C. Kraemer, Ph.D. (Stanford University) is statistical and design consultant. The OSEP/DOE Principal Collaborator is Ellen Schiller, Ph.D. Nilantha Lenora, B.S., is a medical student at George Washington University School of Medicine.

REFERENCES

American Psychiatric Association: Diagnostic and Statistical Manual of Mental Disorders, 3rd Edition. Washington, DC, American Psychiatric Association, 1980

American Psychiatric Association: Diagnostic and Statistical Manual of Mental Disorders, 4th Edition (DSM-IV). Washington, DC, American Psychiatric Association, 1994

Angold A, Costello EJ, Erkanli A: Comorbidity. J Child Psychol Psychiatry 40:57–87, 1999

Beck AT, Ward CH, Mendelsohn M, et al: An inventory for measuring depression. Arch Gen Psychiatry 4:561–571, 1961

Biederman J, Newcorn J, Sprich S: Comorbidity of attention deficit hyperactivity disorder with conduct, depressive, anxiety, and other disorders. Am J Psychiatry 148:564–577, 1991

Biederman J, Faraone SV, Milberger S, et al: Is childhood oppositional defiant disorder a precursor to adolescent conduct disorder? Findings from a four-year follow-up study of children with ADHD. J Am Acad Child Adolesc Psychiatry 35:1193–1204, 1996

Bird H, Gould M, Staghezza-Jaramillo B: The comorbidity of ADHD in a community sample of children aged 6 through 16 years. Journal of Child and Family Studies 3:365–378, 1990

Bird HR, Andrews H, Schwab-Stone M, et al: Global measures of impairment for epidemiologic and clinical use with children and adolescents. Int J Methods Psychiatric Res 6:295–307, 1996

Buitelaar J, Van der Gaag R, Swaab-Barneveld HS, et al: Prediction of clinical response to methylphenidate in children with attention-deficit hyperactivity disorder. J Am Acad Child Adolesc Psychiatry 34:1025–1032, 1995

Cantwell DP: Child psychiatry: introduction and overview, in Comprehensive Textbook of Psychiatry VI. Edited by Kaplan HI, Sadock BJ. Baltimore, MD, Williams & Wilkins, 1995, pp 2151–2154

Conners CK, Epstein J, March JS, et al: Multimodal treatment of ADHD (MTA): an overall measure of treatment outcome. J Am Acad Child Adolesc Psychiatry 40:159–167, 2001

Diamond I, Tannock R, Schachar R: Response to methylphenidate in children with ADHD and comorbid anxiety. J Am Acad Child Adolesc Psychiatry 38:402–409, 1999

DuPaul G, Barkley R, McMurray M: Response of children with ADHD to methylphenidate: interaction with internalizing symptoms. J Am Acad Child Adolesc Psychiatry 33:894–903, 1994

Gresham FM, Elliott SN: Social Skills Rating System—Parent, Teacher and Child Forms. Circle Pines, MN, American Guidance Systems, 1989

Hinshaw, SP: On the distinction between attentional problems/hyperactivity and conduct problems/aggression in child psychopathology. Psychol Bull 101:443–463, 1987

Jensen P, Martin C, Cantwell D: Comorbidity in ADHD: implications for research, practice, and DSM-IV. J Am Acad Child Adolesc Psychiatry 36:1065–1079, 1997

Jensen P*, Rubio-Stipec M*, Dulcan M, et al: The NIMH methods for the epidemiology of child and adolescent mental disorders (MECA) study: are both parent and child informants always needed? J Am Acad Child Adolesc Psychiatry 38(12):1569–1579, 1999 (* designates joint first authorship)

Kovacs M, Beck AT: An empirical-clinical approach toward a definition of childhood depression, in Depression in Childhood. Edited by Schulterbrandt JG, Raskin A. New York: Raven Press, 1977, pp 1–25

Kraemer HC: Statistical issues in assessing comorbidity. Stat Med 14:721–733, 1995

Livingston R, Dykman R, Ackerman P: The frequency and significance of additional self-reported psychiatric diagnoses in children with ADD. J Abnorm Child Psychol 18:465–478, 1990

March JS, Parker JD, Sullivan K, et al: The Multidimensional Anxiety Scale for Children (MASC): factor structure, reliability, and validity. J Am Acad Child Adolesc Psychiatry 36:554–565, 1997

March JS, Swanson JM, Arnold LE, et al: Anxiety as a predictor and outcome variable in the MTA study: analysis using hierarchical linear modeling. J Abnorm Child Psychol 28:527–541, 2000

MTA Cooperative Group: 14-Month randomized clinical trial of treatment strategies for attention deficit hyperactivity disorder. Arch Gen Psychiatry 56(12):1073–1086, 1999a

MTA Cooperative Group: Moderator and mediator challenges to the MTA study: effects of comorbid anxiety disorder, family poverty, session attendance, and community medication on treatment outcome. Arch Gen Psychiatry 56(12):1088–1096, 1999b

Pliszka S: Effect of anxiety on cognition, behavior, and stimulant response in ADHD. J Am Acad Child Adolesc Psychiatry 28:882–887, 1989

Pliszka S: Comorbidity of ADHD and overanxious disorder. J Am Acad Child Adolesc Psychiatry 31:197–203, 1992

Quay H: Classification of the disruptive behavior disorders, in Handbook of Disruptive Behavior Disorders. Edited by Quay HC, Hogan AE. New York, Kluwer Academic/Plenum, 1999, pp 3–21

Robins E, Guze SB: Establishment of diagnostic validity in psychiatric illness: its application to schizophrenia. Am J Psychiatry 126:983–987, 1970

Shaffer D, Fisher P, Dulcan M, et al: The second version of the NIMH Diagnostic Interview Schedule for Children (DISC-2). J Am Acad Child Adolesc Psychiatry 35:865–877, 1996

Swanson JM: School-Based Assessments and Interventions for ADD Students. Irvine, CA, K.C. Publications, 1992

Tannock R, Ickowicz A, Schachar R: Differential effects of methylphenidate on working memory in ADHD children with and without comorbid anxiety. J Am Acad Child Adolesc Psychiatry 34:886–896, 1995

Urman R, Ickowicz A, Fulford P, et al: An exaggerated cardiovascular response to methylphenidate in ADHD children with anxiety. J Child Adolesc Psychopharmacol 5:29–37, 1995

Wechsler D: Wechsler Individual Achievement Test—Manual. San Antonio, TX, The Psychological Corporation, 1992

Wells KC, Epstein JN, Hinshaw SP, et al: Parenting and family stress treatment outcomes in attention-deficit/hyperactivity disorder (ADHD): an empirical analysis in the MTA study. J Abnorm Child Psychol 28:543–553, 2000

Woolston JL, Rosenthal SL, Riddle MA, et al: Childhood comorbidity of anxiety/affective disorders and behavior disorders. J Am Acad Child Adolesc Psychiatry 28:707–713, 1989

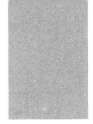

PART IV   EXPLORING ALTERNATIVES

12

Implications of Genetic Epidemiology for Classification

Kathleen R. Merikangas, Ph.D.

The lack of validity of the diagnostic nomenclature is a major impediment to progress in elucidating the etiology of cognitive, emotional, and behavior disorders (Kendell 1989). Advances in neuroscience and genetics that lead to enhanced understanding of the structure and function of the human brain, as well as of the role of genetic and environmental factors involved in cognition, emotion, and behavior, will have a major impact on classification. Likewise, advances in the measurement and observation of the major components of behavior will facilitate identification of etiologic mechanisms. This chapter describes the relevance of advances in genetics of complex diseases for classification and demonstrates the role of genetic epidemiology, in general, and the family study, in particular, in informing classification.

RELEVANCE OF ADVANCES IN GENETICS TO CLASSIFICATION

The announcement that the human genome has now been sequenced has generated widespread excitement about enhanced potential to understand and treat human disease. The characterization of the human genome is expected to facilitate this process so human disease genes may be more rapidly identified (Collins et al. 1998; Watson 1990).

Despite these advances in characterizing human genotypes, application of this knowledge to human diseases is still limited by the complexity of the process through which genes exert their influence. A lack of one-to-one correspondence between the genotype and phenotype is clearly the rule rather than the exception for most human disorders. Phenomena such as *penetrance* (i.e., probability of phenotypic expression among individuals with susceptibility gene), *variable expressivity* (i.e., degree to which susceptible individuals express components of genotype), *gene-environment interaction* (i.e., expression of genotype only in presence of particular environmental exposures), *pleiotropy* (i.e., capacity of gene to manifest simultaneously several different phenotypes), and *genetic heterogeneity* (i.e., different genes leading to indistinguishable phenotypes) have been demonstrated for several human disorders for which susceptibility genes have been identified.

Two of these phenomena that have been of particular concern for genetic nosology are **genetic heterogeneity**, or *one from many*, and **pleiotropy**, or *many from one*. These two situations are reflected in the nosologic tension between lumping and splitting, as described by Victor McKusick (1973) in his review of historical developments in genetic nosology. With increasing specialization within medicine, there has been a tendency to split categories excessively. The lumpers have corrected the oversplitting, but advances in genetics have led to a new wave of "better founded splitting," based on increased ability to detect subtler phenotypically similar but genotypically heterogeneous conditions.

Marfan syndrome is a classic example of pleiotropy. The genetic mutation causing Marfan syndrome has now been identified as fibrillin I on chromosome 15 (Child 1997). The diagnostic criteria for Marfan syndrome based on clinical signs require one of the following five conditions: lens dislocation, aortic dilatation or dissection, dural ectasia, skeletal features, and one other affected system (De Paepe et al. 1996). A single mutation in the genes involved in the production of connective tissue leads to manifestations across multiple organ systems.

Breast cancer provides an illustration of genetic heterogeneity, another basic nosologic problem in genetics. Although family study research is beginning to examine differences in breast cancer among those with and without particular gene markers, the basic breast cancer phenotype has not been adequately differentiated (Szabo and King 1997). Patterns of comorbidity with other cancers and sex differences have been valuable in discriminating different genetic forms of breast cancer (King et al. 1993). Table 12-1 shows that different familial types of breast cancer have different genetic alleles. Whereas families with predominantly affected females or those with both breast and ovarian cancer are more likely to have the

TABLE 12-1   Genetic heterogeneity (BRCA mutations) and breast cancer

Family group	N	BRCA1	BRCA2	Other
No males	211	0.55	0.26	0.19
Male breast	26	0.16	0.76	0.08
Breast/ovarian	94	0.81	0.14	0.05
Female breast	117	0.26	0.32	0.42
All families	237	0.52	0.32	0.16

Source.   Adapted from Ford et al. 1998.

breast cancer locus 1 (BRCA1) mutation (Ford et al. 1998) listed, families with male breast cancer primarily arise from the breast cancer locus 2 (BRCA2) mutation (Miki et al. 1994). Thus, sex differences in recurrence risk and comorbidity across cancer types may be used to identify more homogeneous forms of cancer.

GENE–ENVIRONMENT INTERACTION

Gene–environment interaction characterizes a broad range of human diseases such as cancer and birth defects. The classic examples of gene–environment interaction are the inborn errors of metabolism, such as phenylketonuria, that manifest only when susceptible individuals are exposed to a particular protein or exogenous substance. Glucose-6-phosphate-dehydrogenase (G6PD) deficiency, an X-linked disorder caused by mutation on the long arm of the X chromosome, is another illustration of gene–environment interaction. The expression of this disorder becomes manifest as hemolytic anemia only when the susceptible individual is exposed to certain drugs or fava beans (Cavalli-Sforza and Bodmer 1971). Birth defects have also been found to result from gene–environment interaction. For example, Hwang et al. (1995) assessed the effects of the interaction between maternal cigarette smoking and a transforming growth factor alpha (TGFA) polymorphism on the risk for oral clefts. Oral clefts were increased only among women with the TaqI polymorphism who smoked (Khoury 1997a). Likewise, many forms of cancer such as retinoblastoma (Vogel 1979) arise from somatic mutations to the second allele among individuals who carry a susceptibility allele at a particular locus. Not only is the expression of genes modified by the environment, but there also is now substantial evidence to indicate that numerous environmental factors may actually alter the genotype, as is characteristic of many forms of cancer. Genes may also be involved in the response or resistance to purely environmental agents such as diet, stress, exercise, drugs, and nutritional deficiencies

(Omenn and Motulsky 1978; Risch et al. 1995). The methods of genetic epidemiology are designed specifically to identify gene–environment interactions (Ottman 1995; Yang and Khoury 1997).

Alzheimer's disease (AD) provides an excellent model of a disease with both genetic heterogeneity and gene–environment interaction. There are some major autosomal dominant genes for early-onset familial AD with extremely high relative and absolute risk (Slooter and van Duijn 1997). However, such genes are very rare in the population and have little public health significance. In contrast, there is increasing evidence that the apolipoprotein E (Apo E) E4 allele is associated with both late-onset familial AD and the more common sporadic AD (Corder et al. 1993; Slooter and van Duijn 1997; Tsai et al. 1994). Among families at high risk for late-onset AD, disease risk has been shown to increase with the number of E4 alleles (Corder et al. 1993; Saunders et al. 1993). Finally, environmental risk, such as head injuries and anti-inflammatory agents, has been shown to interact with the Apo E genotypes to protect against or potentiate development of AD (Mayeux et al. 1998).

Therefore, the lack of validity of diagnostic categories is by no means unique to psychiatry. Similar to other domains of complex disorders, the major impediments to the establishment of validity of the classification of psychiatric disorders are the unreliability of measurement (of both diagnoses and markers), the lack of specificity of risk factors and biological markers, and the lack of one-to-one correspondence between the phenotype and genotype, likely attributable to both etiologic and phenotypic heterogeneity and gene–environment interaction (Merikangas 1999). The earlier-cited examples of complex etiology for diseases with well-defined phenotypes and known genetic etiology highlight the importance of simultaneous application of systematic research on the classification of the psychiatric disorders as well as on their pathogenesis. As the tools of molecular biology, genetics, and neuroimaging uncover etiologic processes, the application of family study and longitudinal research may assist in the refinement of phenotypic heterogeneity. The following section describes the goals, methods, and examples of the family study method to refine psychiatric classification.

APPLICATION OF FAMILY STUDY DATA TO CLASSIFICATION

Background

There is consistent evidence that nearly all the psychiatric disorders are familial and that genetic factors account for a significant proportion of the variance in their etiology. In fact, controlled studies have revealed that a family history is the most potent and consistent risk factor for the development of most of the major psychiatric disorders (Merikangas and Swendsen 1997). The classic application of family studies was to test adherence to Mendelian patterns of transmission. Family studies also provide estimates of recurrence risk as a function of population prevalence (λ), an important precondition for determining the power of linkage and association studies (Risch 1990). Whereas λ tends to exceed 20 for most autosomal dominant diseases and those for which the genetic basis has been identified, the range of values of λ derived from family studies of migraine, for example, tends to range from 2 to 3. In general, there is an inverse relationship between the magnitude of the effect of a gene that contributes to disease susceptibility and the population prevalence because of selective disadvantage. Common diseases are far more likely to result from multiple genes or interactions between several predisposing loci (Risch 1994).

The utility of family study and longitudinal data in informing classification was already evident in the seventeenth century. Sydenham (1848) developed the first disease classification system, which was based on the external symptoms and signs of a disease because the underlying processes were impenetrable at that time. He proposed the following components of disease classification: inclusion criteria, exclusion criteria, outcome criteria, laboratory studies, and family studies. These criteria also form the basis of the often-cited paper on the establishment of the validity of the diagnostic categories (Robins and Guze 1970).

The assumption that within-family similarity is greater than between-family similarity is critical to its application to test nosology. Within-family designs minimize the probability of heterogeneity, assuming that the etiology of a disease is likely to be homotypic within families. This design reduces or eliminates the danger of genetic heterogeneity, which has been a major impediment to progress in psychiatry. Family studies can be employed to study the validity of diagnostic categories by assessing the specificity of transmission of symptom patterns and disorders *within* as compared with *between* families (Smoller and Tsuang 1998; Tsuang et al. 1993). Family study data may be employed to examine modes of disease transmission, reduce heterogeneity, identify the phenotypic signal (i.e., core features, subtypes, thresholds, boundaries/overlap with other syndromes), and evaluate mechanisms for comorbidity. Twin studies provide an even more powerful approach to resolving classification issues because they can distinguish genetic from environmental similarity within families.

In general, the family study method and its extension to other types of relatives, including twins, has been grossly underutilized for psychiatric and behavioral phenotypes. In a series of papers on diverse disorders, Kendler et al. (1992, 1993, 1995, 1996) have investigated a range of issues of relevance to psychiatric classification: the definitions of depression (Kendler et al. 1992, 1996), comorbidity between major depression and phobias (Kendler et al. 1993), and common genetic and environmental factors underlying a variety of psychiatric syndromes (Kendler et al. 1995). Twin studies have also been employed to examine operational definitions of schizophrenia (McGuffin et al. 1984), and subtypes and sex differences in substance abuse (Pickens et al. 1995). Finally, family studies have been employed to distinguish between disease subtypes and overlapping syndromes (e.g., Maier and Merikangas 1996; Maier et al. 1993, 1994; Merikangas 1990; Merikangas et al. 1994; Skre et al. 1994). The following section describes some examples of the application of family study data to resolve nosologic issues.

Examples of Nosologic Implications of Family Study Data

The Yale Family Study of Comorbidity of Substance Use Disorders and Psychopathology was designed specifically to examine sources of comorbidity, and to resolve thresholds and boundaries of the affective disorders and substance use disorders (Merikangas et al. 1998, 1999). Examples of specific questions involving classification that have been examined in the Yale Family Study include the specificity of diagnostic subtypes, sex differences in diagnostic thresholds, and sources of comorbidity between diagnostic entities.

Specificity of Diagnostic Subtypes

To test the distinction between alcohol abuse and dependence introduced in the DSM-III (American Psychiatric Association 1980), familial patterns of expression of alcohol abuse and dependence were examined. The results revealed that the prevalence of alcohol abuse was similar among relatives of probands with alcohol abuse or dependence compared with those of psychiatric and nonpsychiatric control subjects. In contrast, relatives of probands with alcohol dependence had increased lifetime prevalence rates of alcohol dependence (Merikangas et al. 1998a). This confirms the validity of the distinction between alcohol abuse and dependence.

The tendency for anxiety disorders to co-occur within individuals has been well established in population-based studies (Wittchen et al. 1994). The family study method may be employed to examine the specificity of familial aggregation of the subtypes of anxiety. Data from the Yale Family Study reveal that the subtypes of anxiety tend to breed true in these families. That is, relatives of probands with panic disorder have elevated

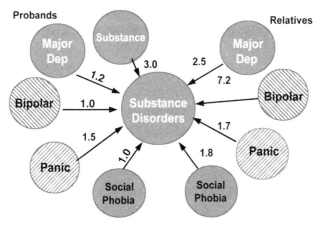

FIGURE 12-1   Adjusted risk ratios of substance disorders in relatives.

rates of panic disorder, and relatives of probands with social phobia have elevated rate of social phobia compared with each other, as well as compared
with relatives of control subjects without anxiety disorders (Figure 12-1;
Merikangas and Stevens 1998; Merikangas et al. 1998a). Thus, despite
the high magnitude of overlap between the subtypes of anxiety disorders
within individuals, these disorders tend to aggregate independently in families. Fyer et al. (1995) showed that simple phobia and social phobia also
tend to cluster independently in families. Likewise, there was familial
specificity of the drug of preference in a family study of substance use
disorders (Merikangas et al. 1998b).

Specificity of Biological Markers
One of the major impediments to the application of family, twin, and high-
risk study data to classification is the lack of inclusion of multiple psychiatric comparison groups within particular studies. Multiple comparison
groups enable discrimination of specificity of biological or clinical phenomena. Although most studies of biological markers yield differences
between the relatives of psychiatric probands compared with control subjects, comparison across studies reveals that the markers may be associated
with many different psychiatric disorders. This lack of specificity is not
likely to lead to information for further genetic studies.

The above-cited high-risk study of comorbidity of anxiety disorders and
alcoholism revealed different patterns of potentiated startle among offspring of parents with anxiety disorders compared with offspring of alcoholic parents and control subjects (Grillon et al. 1997). The findings reveal
that children of alcoholic parents differ from both children of parents with
anxiety disorders and control subjects, thereby suggesting specificity of

the finding of enhanced prepulse inhibition of the startle reflex among off-spring of alcoholic probands. Such studies will be increasingly important in studying the impact of genetic vulnerability factors and in identifying environmental factors that may mediate genetic expression.

Family study data may also be employed to examine whether there is a dose–response effect in recurrence risk among offspring as a function of the number of affected parents. Offspring of two affected parents have a twofold risk of anxiety disorders compared with offspring of one affected parent, and offspring of one affected parent have a twofold increased risk of anxiety compared with those of couples with neither parent affected (Merikangas et al. 1999). In contrast, no dose–response effect was observed for depression for which there was a main effect of parental depression on rates of offspring depression; however, there was no elevation in risk among offspring of dually affected couples compared with those in which only one parent had depression (Dierker et al. 1999). Likewise, conduct disorder in offspring was associated with psychopathology in both parents, irrespective of the specific form of psychiatric disorder expressed in the parents (Dierker et al. 1999; Merikangas et al. 1998d). This *lack* of specificity suggests that factors attributable to general familial maladaptation are associated with parental concordance rather than with specific factors associated with specific disorders. In this situation, disease-specific genetic factors would be less likely to underlie disorders among offspring than those with some evidence of specificity.

Causes of Comorbidity

Family study methods have also been employed to examine mechanisms for comorbidity. As shown below, evidence for shared pathophysiology in family studies would be derived from an increase in rates of the comorbid disorder (and *not* the index disorder) in the relatives of probands with only the index disorder, as compared with those among control subjects. Similarly, in twin studies, increased rates of the comorbid disorder in the co-twins of monozygotic probands, as compared with dizygotic probands with only the index disorder, would support shared pathophysiology. Alternatively, if the comorbid disorder is elevated among the relatives of probands with the "pure" index disorder, but only when coupled with the index disorder, then an etiologic model would be more likely to explain the association (Merikangas 1990; Merikangas and Stevens 1998).

Family studies by Merikangas et al. (1994) and Maier and colleagues (Maier and Merikangas 1996; Maier et al. 1993, 1994) investigated the familial patterns of comorbidity among affective disorders, anxiety disorders, and alcoholism. Patterns of cosegregation of alcoholism, depression, and anxiety disorders among relatives of probands with each of these conditions as compared with control subjects suggested some degree of shared susceptibility factors for alcoholism, panic, and depression, based on an elevated risk of alcoholism among the relatives of probands with pure panic disorder. A subsequent family study was designed to examine familial patterns of comorbidity according to the specific subtypes of anxiety and substance abuse among probands and relatives (Merikangas and Stevens 1998; Merikangas et al. 1998a). The results are shown in Figure 12-1. Disorders among the probands are shown on the left side of the figure, the major outcome of substance disorders among the relatives is shown in the middle of the figure, and comorbid disorders among relatives are shown on the right side of the figure. The adjusted risk ratios for the association between proband disorders with substance dependence in the relatives are shown above each arrow. All of the risk ratios were controlled for proband and relative comorbidity; proband sex and diagnostic selection group; and the age, sex, and interview status of the relative. These results reveal that panic disorder, major depression, and substance use disorders result in part from shared familial risk factors because there was an elevation in the risk ratios for the association between these disorders in probands with substance use disorders in relatives. By contrast, the lack of an association between proband social phobia and bipolar disorder with substance use disorders in relatives is consistent with a causal link between the latter disorders with substance use disorders in relatives. The importance of characterizing probands and relatives according to the *subtype* of anxiety, depression, and substance use disorder is illustrated by these findings.

FUTURE DIRECTIONS IN CLASSIFICATION

Role of Genetic Epidemiology

The methods of genetic epidemiology will be essential to harvest the fruits of progress achieved by identifying the human genome and its protein products (summarized in Table 12-2). As our tools for measuring phenotypes become more sophisticated, information on clinical signs and symptoms may be combined with that designed to penetrate the brain processes

TABLE 12-2   Applications of genetic epidemiology

■ Examine modes of transmission in family and twin studies.
■ Reduce genetic heterogeneity.
■ Identify phenotypic signal (i.e., core features, subtypes, thresholds).
■ Evaluate mechanisms for comorbidity.
■ Examine association between diseases and genetic markers.
■ Estimate prevalence and attributable risk of genetic markers.
■ Identify specific environmental risk factors that interact
   with genetic markers (i.e., genetic case-control studies).

underlying behavioral phenotypes. Family study data will have an increasingly important role in refining phenotypic heterogeneity and, ultimately, in identifying clinical manifestations of genetically heterogeneous conditions. Application of family and twin study data to evaluate core features, subtypes, thresholds, and boundaries and overlap between disorders will form an essential foundation for mapping disease genes.

A second application of genetic epidemiology essential for progress is the recruitment of population-based samples of families. Current knowledge regarding the distribution of disease genes derives from families with multiply affected members. However, such families may not be representative of the general population. Currently, much of the ongoing clinical genetic research is not population based, and much of population-based epidemiological research does not assess genetic risk factors. For example, the risk of breast cancer attributable to BRCA1 in the general population is unknown because current information is based solely on families of affected probands (Corder et al. 1993). Therefore, population-based epidemiological studies are increasingly needed to quantify the impact of gene variants on the risk of disease, death, and disability (Steinberg et al. 1997). Increased information on population frequencies of genes will also enhance the power of association studies using case-control designs (Risch and Merikangas 1996; Schaid and Somer 1993).

A third area of relevance of genetic epidemiology is the identification of environmental modifiers of vulnerability genes. Epidemiology has traditionally focused on the definition and measurement of environmental risk factors, particularly for infectious diseases. In psychiatry, there has been far less progress in identifying environmental risk factors, particularly with specificity for the development of particular forms of psychopathology. For emotional, cognitive, and behavioral disorders, there are some interesting models that may provide evidence of interactions between environmental and genetic or biological risk factors. Some examples of interactions between biological and environmental vulnerability factors include the following:

- Susceptibility genes seem to be necessary but not sufficient for the development of schizophrenia (Tienari et al. 1994; Wahlberg et al. 1997).
- Alcoholism in adoptees results from interaction between a biological background and environmental exposure to alcoholism (Cutrona et al. 1994).
- Behaviorally inhibited temperament appears to be protective against the development of conduct problems (Kagan 1994).
- Childhood minor physical anomalies predict psychiatric status 10 years later only in the presence of environmental risk (Pine et al. 1997).

Linking the Genotype and Phenotype

Advances in neuroscience have also enhanced our ability to measure human brain structure and function. This should ultimately lead to better characterization of the components of cognition, emotion, and behavior that underlie the major psychiatric disorders. It is essential to integrate progress in defining and measuring psychiatric phenotypes with advances in identifying the genetic basis of human higher order functioning. At present, knowledge of a particular gene does not permit prediction of the phenotype, nor does knowledge of a phenotype permit inferences regarding the genotype, particularly for the components of disorders relevant to psychiatry. Therefore, successful identification of the joint impact of genetic and environmental risk factors will require research that spans all levels of the pathways between the genotype and phenotype.

The complex links between the genotype and phenotype are depicted in Figure 12-2. The future calls for increasing collaboration across multiple disciplines, using all available tools to address etiologic questions. Greater understanding of etiologic processes will enhance prevention and intervention efforts. Genetic epidemiology will play a major role in refining the phenotype, identifying homogeneous disease subtypes, estimating population prevalence of genetic markers, and identifying environmental exposures involved in gene-environment interactions (Khoury 1997). Data generated from such collaborations are urgently needed for the development of effective interventions and public health policy.

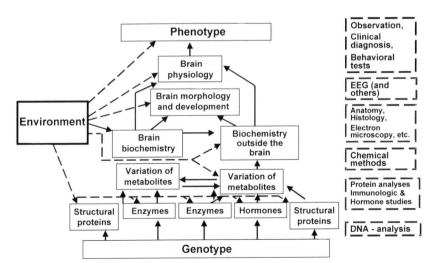

FIGURE 12-2   Complex links between genotype and phenotype.
Source. Adapted from Vogel and Motulsky 1995.

REFERENCES

American Psychiatric Association: Diagnostic and Statistical Manual of Mental Disorders, 3rd Edition. Washington, DC, American Psychiatric Association, 1980

Cavalli-Sforza LL, Bodmer WF: Chapter 12, in The Genetics of Human Populations. San Francisco, CA, W.H. Freeman, 1971, p 756

Child AH: Marfan syndrome—current medical and genetic knowledge: how to treat and when. J Card Surg 12(suppl 2):131–136, 1997

Collins FS, Patrinos A, Jordan E, et al: New goals for the US Human Genome Project. Science 282:682–689, 1998

Corder EH, Saunders AM, Strittmatter WJ, et al: Gene dose of apolipoprotein E type 4 allele and the risk of Alzheimer's disease in late onset families. Science 261:921–923, 1993

Cutrona CE, Cadoret RJ, Suhr JA, et al: Interpersonal variables in the prediction of alcoholism among adoptees: evidence for gene-environment interactions. Compr Psychiatry 35:171–179, 1994

De Paepe A, Devereux TB, Dietz HC, et al: Revised diagnostic criteria for Marfan syndrome. Am J Med Genet 62:417–426, 1996

Dierker LC, Merikangas KR, Szatmari P: The influence of parental diagnostic concordance on risk for psychopathology in offspring. J Am Acad Child Adolesc Psychiatry 38(3):280–288, 1999

Ford D, Easton DF, Bishop DT, et al: Risks of cancer in BRCA1-mutation carriers. Breast Cancer Linkage Consortium. Am J Hum Genet 56:265–71, 1998

Fyer AJ, Mannuzza S, Chapman TF, et al: Specificity of familial aggregation of phobic disorders. Arch Gen Psychiatry 52:564–573, 1995

Grillon C, Dierker L, Merikangas KR: Startle modulation in children at risk for anxiety disorders and/or alcoholism. J Am Acad Child Adolesc Psychiatry 36:925–932, 1997

Hwang SJ, Beaty TH, Panny SR, et al: Association study of transforming growth factor alpha TaqI polymorphisms and oral clefts: indication of gene-environment interaction in a population-based sample of infants with birth defects. Am J Epidemiol 141:629–636, 1995

Kagan J: Galen's Prophecy: Temperament in Human Nature. Boulder, CO, Westview Press, 1994

Kendell RE: Clinical validity. Psychol Med 19:45–55, 1989

Kendler KS, Neale MC, Kessler RC, et al: A population-based twin study of major depression in women: the impact of varying definitions of illness. Arch Gen Psychiatry 49:257–266, 1992

Kendler KS, Neale MC, Kessler RC, et al: Major depression and phobias: the genetic and environmental sources of comorbidity. Psychol Med 23:361–371, 1993

Kendler K, Walters E, Neale M, et al: The structure of the genetic and environmental risk factors for six major psychiatric disorders in women. Arch Gen Psychiatry 52:374–383, 1995

Kendler KS, Eaves LJ, Walters EE, et al: The identification and validation of distinct depressive syndromes in a population-based sample of female twins. Arch Gen Psychiatry 53:391–399, 1996

Khoury M: Genetic epidemiology and the future of disease prevention and public health. Epidemiol Rev 19:175–180, 1997

Khoury MJ, Wagener DK: An epidemiologic evaluation of the use of genetics to improve the predictive value of disease risk factors. Am J Hum Genet 56:835–844, 1995

King MC, Rowell S, Love SM: Inherited breast and ovarian cancer: what are the risks? what are the choices? JAMA 269:1975–1980, 1993

Maier W, Merikangas K: Co-occurrence and co-transmission of affective disorders and alcoholism in families. Br J Psychiatry 168:93–100, 1996

Maier W, Minges J, Lichtermann D: Alcoholism and panic disorder: co-occurrence and co-transmission in families. Eur Arch Psychiatry Clin Neurosci 243:205–211, 1993

Maier W, Lichtermann D, Minges J: The relationship of alcoholism and unipolar depression: a controlled family study. Psychiatr Res 28:303–317, 1994

Mayeux R, Saunders A, Shea S, et al: Utility of the apolipoprotein E genotype in the diagnosis of Alzheimer's disease. N Engl J Med 338:506–511, 1998

McGuffin P, Farmer AE, Gottesman II: Twin concordance for operationally defined schizophrenia: confirmation of familiality and heritability. Arch Gen Psychiatry 41:541–545, 1984

McKusick VA: The nosology of genetic diseases, in Medical Genetics. Edited by McKusick VA, Claiborne R. New York, HP Publishing, 1973, pp 211–220

Merikangas KR: Comorbidity for anxiety and depression: a review of family and genetic studies, in Comorbidity of Mood and Anxiety Disorders. Edited by Maser JD, Cloninger CR. Washington, DC, American Psychiatric Press, 1990, pp 331–348

Merikangas KR: Editorial: the next decade of psychiatric epidemiology. Int J Methods Psychol Res 8:1–5, 1999

Merikangas KR, Stevens DE: Models of transmission of substance use and comorbid psychiatric disorders, in Dual Diagnosis and Treatment: Substance Abuse and Comorbid Medical and Psychiatric Disorders. Edited by Kranzler HR, Rounsaville BJ. New York, Marcel Dekker, 1998, pp 31–53

Merikangas KR, Swendsen J: The genetic epidemiology of psychiatric disorders. Epidemiol Rev 19:1–12, 1997

Merikangas KR, Risch N, Weissman M, et al: Comorbidity and co-transmission of alcoholism, anxiety, and depression. Psychol Med 24:69–80, 1994

Merikangas KR, Stevens DE, Fenton B, et al: Co-morbidity and familial aggregation of alcoholism and anxiety disorders. Psychol Med 28:773–788, 1998a

Merikangas KR, Stolar M, Stevens DE, et al: Familial transmission of substance use disorders. Arch Gen Psychiatry 55:973–979, 1998b

Merikangas K, Dierker L, Szatmari P: Psychopathology among offspring of parents with substance abuse and/or anxiety disorders: a high risk study. J Child Psychol Psychiatry 39:711–720, 1998c

Merikangas KR, Avenevoli S, Dierker LC, et al: Vulnerability factors among children at risk for anxiety disorders. Biol Psychiatry 46:1523–1535, 1999

Miki Y, Swensen J, Shattuck-Eidens D, et al: A strong candidate for the breast and ovarian cancer susceptibility gene BRCA1. Science 266:66–76, 1994

Omenn GS, Motulsky AG: Ecogenetics: genetic variation in susceptibility to environmental agents, in Genetic Issues in Public Health and Medicine. Edited by Cohen BH, Lilienfeld AM, Huang PC. Springfield, IL, Thomas, 1978, pp 83–111

Ottman R: Gene-environment interaction and public health. Am J Hum Genet 56:821–823, 1995

Pickens RW, Svikis DS, McGue M, et al: Common genetic mechanisms in alcohol, drug, and mental disorder comorbidity. Drug Alcohol Depend 39:129–138, 1995

Pine D, Shaffer D, Schonfeld I, et al: Minor physical anomalies: modifiers of environmental risks for psychiatric impairment. J Am Acad Child Adolesc Psychiatry 36:395–403, 1997

Risch A, Wallace DM, Bathers S, et al: Slow N-acetylation genotype is a susceptibility factor in occupational and smoking related bladder cancer. Hum Mol Genet 4:231–236, 1995

Risch N: Linkage strategies for genetically complex traits. I. Multilocus models. Am J Hum Genet 46:222–228, 1990

Risch N: Mapping genes for psychiatric disorders, in Genetic Approaches to Mental Disorders. Edited by Gershon ES, Cloninger CR. Washington, DC, American Psychiatric Press, 1994, pp 47–61

Risch N, Merikangas K: The future of genetic studies of complex human diseases. Science 273:1516–1517, 1996

Robins E, Guze SB: Establishment of diagnostic validity in psychiatric illness: its application to schizophrenia. Am J Psychiatry 126:983–987, 1970

Saunders AM, Strittmatter WJ, Schmechel D, et al: Association of the apolipoprotein E allele E4 with late-onset familial and sporadic Alzheimer's disease. Neurology 43:1467–1472, 1993

Schaid DJ, Somer SS: Genotype relative risks: methods for design and analysis of candidate-gene association studies. Am J Hum Genet 53:1114–1126, 1993

Skre I, Onstad S, Edvardsen J, et al: A family study of anxiety disorders: Familial transmission and relationship to mood disorder and psychoactive substance use disorder. Acta Psychiatr Scand 90:366–374, 1994

Slooter A, van Duijn C: Genetic epidemiology of Alzheimer disease. Epidemiol Rev 19(1):107–119, 1997

Smoller JW, Tsuang M: Panic and phobic anxiety: defining phenotypes for genetic studies. Am J Psychiatry 155:1152–1162, 1998

Steinberg KK, Sanderlin KC, Ou C-Y, et al: DNA banking in epidemiologic studies. Epidemiol Rev 19:156–162, 1997

Sydenham T: The Works of Thomas Sydenham. Translated by WA Greenhill. London, England, Sydenham Society, 1848

Szabo C, King MC: Population genetics of BRCA1 and BRCA2. Am J Hum Genet 60:1013–1020, 1997

Tsai MS, Tangalos EG, Petersen RC, et al: Apolipoprotein E: risk factor for Alzheimer disease. Am J Hum Genet 54:643–649, 1994

Tienari P, Wynne LC, Moring J, et al: The Finnish adoptive family study of schizophrenia. Implications for family research. Br J Psychiatry 164(Suppl 23):20–26, 1994

Tsuang MT, Faraone SV, Lyons MJ: Identification of the phenotype in psychiatric genetics. Eur Arch Psychiatry Clin Neurosci 243:131–142, 1993

Vogel F: Genetics of retinoblastoma. Hum Genet 52:1–54, 1979

Vogel F, Motulsky AG: Human Genetics: Problems and Approaches, 2nd Edition. Berlin, Germany, Springer-Verlag, 1995

Wahlberg KE, Wynne LC, Oja H, et al: Gene-environment interaction in vulnerability to schizophrenia: findings from the Finnish Adoptive Family Study of Schizophrenia. Am J Psychiatry 154:355–362, 1997

Watson JD: The human genome project: past, present, and future. Science 248:44–49, 1990

Wittchen HU, Zhao S, Kessler RC, et al: DSM-III-R generalized anxiety disorder in the National Comorbidity Survey. Arch Gen Psychiatry 51:355–364, 1994

Yang Q, Khoury MJ: Evolving Methods in Genetic Epidemiology, III: gene-environment interaction in epidemiologic research. Epidemiol Rev 19:33–43, 1997

13

Importance of Phenotype Definition in Genetic Studies of Child Psychopathology

James J. Hudziak, M.D.

A major obstacle to identifying risk genes for psychiatric conditions is the issue of phenotypic definition. Put simply, if subjects included in psychiatric genetic studies are not correctly selected, the outcome of the study (i.e., to correctly identify genes that may influence the development of the disorder) will be in doubt. Other researchers (e.g., State et al. 2000; Tsuang et al. 1993) have expertly described the impact of polygenic inheritance, incomplete penetrance, variable phenotypic expression, novel molecular genetic mechanisms, and genetic heterogeneity on identifying genetic and environmental risk factors for common conditions of comorbidity on phenotype selection.

This chapter discusses the issue of phenotype selection in genetic studies of common child psychiatric illness. To improve our ability to identify genetic risk factors, child psychiatry will be dependent on the creation of a taxonomic approach that facilitates the correct selection of subjects for gene finding studies. Furthermore, we will need to develop thoughtful

Portions of this chapter appear in Hudziak JJ: "The Role of Phenotypes (Diagnoses) in Genetic Studies of Attention-Deficit Hyperactivity Disorder and Related Child Psychopathology." *Child and Adolescent Psychiatric Clinics of North America* 10:279–298, 2001. Used with permission.

ways to measure environmental and developmental influences on these phenotypes. This is particularly true for the field of child psychiatry, where selecting subjects for genetic studies is complicated by the age of the subject (should the same criteria be used for 2-year-olds as for 15-year-olds?), the gender of the subject (should the same criteria be used for boys and girls?), who the informant is (should mother, father, teacher, subject, or sibling reports be used?), the variable environments to which the subject is exposed (should socioeconomic status, family constellation, and history of trauma be used as modifying environmental variables?), and even the diagnostic approach that is used (should genetic studies on children be conducted using categorical approaches such as DSM, quantitative, or both?).

GENETIC NOSOLOGY FOR CHILD PSYCHIATRIC STUDIES

As Tsuang and colleagues (1993) pointed out,

> For many psychiatric disorders we have a strong foundation of genetic epidemiological data that posits genes as etiological agents. Upon this foundation, the new tools of molecular and statistical genetics promise to build an enduring theoretical and empirical structure that will house solutions to many questions of etiology, pathophysiology, diagnosis, and treatment. (p. 131)

Tsuang et al. also suggested that

> Statistical procedures and molecular genetic techniques have attained a fine degree of resolution. Their ability to find disease genes has revolutionized medicine and raised hopes for breakthroughs in psychiatry. However, such breakthroughs may require an equally discriminating psychiatric nosology—a nomenclature that can more validly discriminate genetic and non-genetic subtypes of illness (and genetic subtypes as well). (p. 139)

Previous research on the genetics of child psychopathology [particularly attention-deficit hyperactivity disorder (ADHD)] has shown that studies are complicated by the following factors: 1) issues regarding the proper use of multiple informants (*informant variance*), 2) agreement or disagreement between different assessments (*instrument variance*), 3) *development*, 4) *gender*, and 5) *comorbidity*. These issues challenge researchers and clinicians who are trying to identify genes that place children at risk for psychiatric conditions. Each issue is described in detail in the following sections.

Informant Variance

Disagreement between informants can lead to misclassification, which has a profound effect on genetic studies (Tsuang et al. 1993). A multi-informant approach is useful in reducing false positives and false negatives, thereby increasing the likelihood of identifying genes that contribute to the development of child psychiatric disorders (Neale et al. 1992). In most studies of child psychopathology, parental reports are fundamental. However, mothers and fathers do not always agree on their child's behavior (Achenbach 1993). Because informants' reports are based on their experience with the child, the setting where they see the child (e.g., school, home), and their personal characteristics, teachers and parents often disagree. Verhulst et al. (1997) provided an elegant example of the difficulties faced when performing research on child and adolescent psychopathology. In their Dutch epidemiological study of adolescent psychopathology, they found that 21.8% of parents reported on the Diagnostic Interview Schedule for Children, Parent Report, version 3.0 (DISC-P) that their adolescent had a DSM-III-R (American Psychiatric Association 1987) disorder; 21.5% of the adolescents also reported on the Diagnostic Interview Schedule for Children, Child Report, version 3.0 (DISC-C) that they had a DSM-III-R disorder. Yet, parents and adolescents agreed in only 4% of the cases. Relying on a single informant may lead to both false positives and false negatives. Because of the high cost of false positives and false negatives to genetic studies, it is important to use multi-informant assessments to reduce errors. This is not to stipulate that a child must have impairment in all settings as reported by all informants. Different constellations of informant agreement/disagreement may indicate different phenotypes and, ultimately, different genotypes.

Twin studies of child psychopathology have often based estimates of heritability on data from parents. However, parents' assessment of twins may be affected by either rater bias (the tendency to overestimate the similarities of siblings) or parental rater contrast (the tendency to underreport psychopathology in the less affected sibling). Both Goodman and Stevenson (1989a, 1989b) and Sherman et al. (1997a) interpreted their data as suggesting that mothers overestimated the similarity of monozygotic twins and underestimated the similarity of dizygotic twins, which lead to biased heritability estimates (Nadder et al. 1998). Eaves et al. (1997), Hudziak et al. (in review), and Thapar et al. (1995) reported findings consistent with a "parental contrast effect," whereby parents underestimated the degree to which the less affected twin manifested ADHD, which can produce spuriously low heritability estimates.

Despite prior reports suggesting that parents of monozygotic twin pairs may overestimate the similarity of their twins (Sherman et al. 1997a), by modeling rater contrast effects on means as well as on variances and co-variances, Hudziak et al. (in review, 2000) were able to show that these data were consistent with the opposite effect. Instead of rater amplification effects, they reported significant rater contrast effects (the tendency of parents to underestimate problems in one twin if the other had more pronounced problems), especially for parents who were rating monozygotic twins. In other words, when responding to DSM interviews, parents of monozygotic twin pairs appeared to magnify the differences between their twins. This "rater contrast" interpretation more parsimoniously accounts for the observed pattern of reduced means and variances of parental ratings of monozygotic pairs compared with dizygotic pairs, as well as much higher monozygotic than dizygotic correlations than the simple assertion that parents of monozygotic pairs overestimate their similarity because they are "identical."

Researchers have repeatedly shown disagreement between parents, children, and teachers on children's behavior problems. Furthermore, it is clear that differences exist in heritability estimates between parent reports and self-reports from adolescents. For instance, Hudziak et al. (2000) showed that the a^2 for Thought Problems varies by the informant, with parental reports ranging between 0.44 and 0.56. Adolescents' self-report was 0.00, and young adults' self-report was 0.27. Similarly, the a^2 for Aggressive Behavior by parental reports was between 0.52 for boys and 0.60 for girls, but for self-report it varied by gender (0.20 for female adolescents, and 0.55 for males) and by development (0.45 for both genders as young adults; Boomsma et al., in review).

The evidence for significant rater variance and contrast effects reinforces the need to obtain data from multiple informants to identify the most useful raters for twin and other family studies of child psychiatric conditions. The evidence presented for rater contrast effects raises the possibility that parent reports alone are insufficient for phenotypic identification in gene mapping studies. These data support the need for multiple informants and quantitative assessment to increase power for identifying heritable phenotypes.

Instrument Variance

There are numerous ways in which the choice of an assessment instrument can affect estimates of genetic and environmental influence and confound the search for phenotypes in genetic studies. After reviewing research on the biases inherent to self-report and survey methodologies, Schwarz (1999) suggested that, instead of seeing these distortions as errors or limitations, we should accept the advantages afforded by different techniques and use multiple, diverse measures of the construct in question to enhance validity. Behavior genetic research must usually rely on recall instead of observation, so this advice bears heeding because biased measurement will generally bias heritability estimates. Three topics in what Schwarz called the "cognitive aspects of survey methodology" (p. 93) are most germane to instrument variance in psychiatric diagnosis: 1) categorical and quantitative applications, 2) item arrangement, and 3) the comparative merits of questionnaires and interview approaches.

Categories and Continua

As Rutter (1997) succinctly stated, "Psychiatric research continues to be troubled by difficulties in measurement. At one time, many investigators thought that the use of standardized interviews and operationalized criteria for diagnosis would solve the problems, but it is evident that they have not" (p. 785). Misclassification is common in child psychiatric genetic studies. For example, the DSM system assumes that disorders are discrete categories defined by a criterion number of symptoms. Regardless of whether it is applied to a checklist or DSM framework, the categorical approach may not provide quantitative differentiation within disorders—a potentially important weakness for genetic research.

To illustrate, by the *categorical* rules of the DSM-IV (American Psychiatric Association 1994), a child with 12 symptoms of ADHD is considered to be categorically equivalent to one with 18. Furthermore, a child having 5 of 9 symptoms from both inattention and hyperactivity-impulsivity groups, yielding 10 total ADHD symptoms, is considered unaffected because he or she would miss the required cut point by 1 in each category. However, a child with 6 inattention and 4 hyperactivity-impulsivity symptoms—also 10 total—meets diagnostic criteria. The categorical approach limits family, twin, and adoptee studies by dichotomizing subjects while ignoring degree of impairment. Although useful for everyday clinical services, this system may be inadequate for identifying phenotypes useful to psychiatric genetic studies. Quantitative approaches that do not ignore the variation between subjects may offer a more discriminating nosology for genetic studies.

Categories and quantitative differentiation have been examined in phenotypic analyses of twin studies of ADHD.

Using latent class analysis (LCA; see Figure 13-1), Hudziak et al. (1998a) reported that DSM-IV ADHD is best modeled as three separate continua

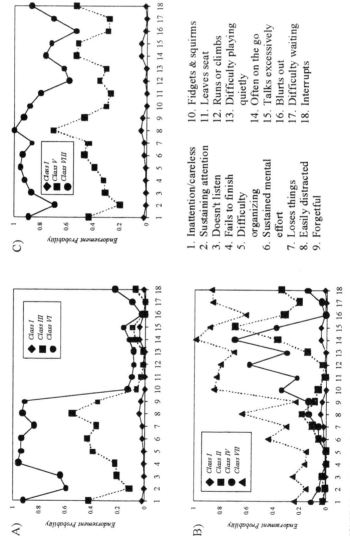

1. Inattention/careless
2. Sustaining attention
3. Doesn't listen
4. Fails to finish
5. Difficulty organizing
6. Sustained mental effort
7. Loses things
8. Easily distracted
9. Forgetful
10. Fidgets & squirms
11. Leaves seat
12. Runs or climbs
13. Difficulty playing quietly
14. Often on the go
15. Talks excessively
16. Blurts out
17. Difficulty waiting
18. Interrupts

FIGURE 13-1 Latent-class analysis of A) primarily inattentive, B) primarily hyperactive, and C) combined type ADHD.

rather than as a discrete disorder—a conclusion shared by Goodman and Stevenson (1989a, 1989b), Levy et al. (1997), and Sherman et al. (1997a)—and reflects a consensus among twin study researchers examining ADHD. However, our same group (Todd et al., in press) demonstrated that there is little evidence for genetic relatedness among the continua. At first, this finding appears counterintuitive, but if we argue that ADHD symptoms exist as continua, then surely the expression of the mild, moderate, and severe forms just represent an example of variable penetrance. Rather, we believe the data indicate that although the symptom criteria for ADHD cluster in apparent severity classes (mild, moderate, and severe), the genetic vulnerability for the classes are distinct. This raises the possibility that different genes influence different levels of attention, hyperactivity, and impulsivity.

In that same population, Hudziak et al. (1999) reported the univariate analysis of Attention Problems symptom count, using a rater contrast model, and found large additive genetic influence (a^2) of 94%, moderate nonshared environmental influence (e^2) of 6%, no shared environmental influence (c^2), and a zygosity specific rater contrast effect of -0.29 for monozygotic and -0.12 for dizygotic pairs. For the Hyperactivity-Impulsivity Problems symptom count domain, a^2 was 93%, e^2 was 7%, and c^2 was 0%. Zygosity-specific rater contrast effects were -0.22 for monozygotic and -0.08 for dizygotic pairs. These high heritability estimates result in part from explicit modeling of error variance (i.e., they are corrected for measurement error). For the bivariate analysis of DSM-IV ADHD as symptom counts from the Attention Problems and Hyperactivity-Impulsivity Problems domains, we obtained substantial estimates of additive genetic variance (94% for Attention Problems, 93% for Hyperactivity-Impulsivity Problems), with a modest but significant genetic correlation between the two domains (genetic correlation of 43%).

These results strongly support the conclusions of Sherman et al. (1997a, 1997b), whose analyses of parent and teacher rating data in their study of DSM-III-R ADHD led them to conclude "that genetic factors are etiologically important in the expression of the separate dimensions of ADHD and the covariation between them" (Sherman et al. 1997a, p. 745). Taken together with the results from the latent class and factor analysis of ADHD, these data also support the findings of Levy et al. (1997), who studied DSM-III-R ADHD in Australian twins and concluded that "ADHD is best viewed as the extreme of a behavior that varies genetically throughout the entire population" (p. 737). Unlike Levy et al., recent findings indicate that this taxonomic variability is due in part to discrete genetic influences (Hudziak et al. 2000).

Item Arrangement

Item order alone can have a powerful effect on diagnostic survey results. Knowles and Byers (1996) showed that respondents' endorsements tend to be more polarized when they are shown in a group of related items and independent of the content of a question. Clustering items exposes the test giver's assumptions about (in our case) the disease underlying a list of symptoms (Schwarz 1999). After sensing the relationship between items, an informant may skew his or her responses to the later symptoms so they "fit" with earlier answers. In addition, consistent responses to the first few items may cause the "mindlessness" described by Langer and Imber (1980), which leads to careless and systematically biased reports, particularly to the later items in a list. Because most DSM interview protocols query symptoms grouped by diagnostic category, they may be sensitive to item-order context effects. However, for twin research, informants who are comparing the twins and either inflating or minimizing differences in their behavior compound the limitations of interviews. This biases their ratings and the heritability estimates derived from them. In fact, some interview instructions (e.g., the Child and Adolescent Psychiatric Assessment [CAPA]) encourage direct comparison to other children without discouraging within-family comparisons. In an analysis of DSM-IV interview responses by twins' parents, evidence was found for this sort of rater contrast effect (Hudziak et al., in review). Using the same large general population sample of adolescent female twins, we performed genetic analysis to determine the heritability of symptom domains when treated as continuous measures or as DSM-IV categorical subtypes. In addition to exploring categories versus continua, we attempted to correct for parent rater contrast by model fitting to derive adjusted estimates of the heritabilities of attention and hyperactivity-impulsivity domains.

In analyses of DSM-IV ADHD categorical subtypes, approximately 7% of subjects met DSM-IV criteria for one of the three types of ADHD. We also found that these subtypes were highly heritable, with additive genetic influences accounting for 87% of the variance in risk of Attention Problems (prevalence of 4.0%), 71% of the variance in risk of Hyperactivity-Impulsivity Problems (prevalence of 0.8%), and 93% of the variance in risk of Combined Type (prevalence of 2.2%). There was little or no evidence for shared environmental influence and modest nonshared environmental influence (5% for Attention, 12% for Hyperactivity-Impulsivity, and 3% for Combined Type). The most parsimonious model included a zygosity-dependent rater contrast effect (the tendency for parents to diminish the magnitude of the symptoms in the less affected twin), which was greater for parents of monozygotic pairs (−0.25 for Attention, −0.013 for Hyperactivity-Impulsivity, and −0.19 for Combined Type) than for dizygotic pairs (−0.07 for Attention, −0.01 for Hyperactivity-Impulsivity, and −0.10 for Combined Type). In the genetic analyses of categorical subtypes, both model-fitting and logistic regression approaches confirmed highly significant evidence for genetic effects on Attention and Combined-Type subtypes. However, perhaps because of the low overall lifetime prevalence of (0.8%), in the case of Hyperactivity-Impulsivity, the hypothesis of no genetic influence could not be rejected. The loss of statistical power associated with the genetic analysis of categorical traits of low prevalence (c.f., Neale et al. 1994) was such that 95% confidence intervals for the shared environmental variance were as high as 32% of the variance for Attention Problems, 37% for Combined Type, and 80% for Hyperactivity-Impulsivity Problems. Furthermore, using categorical assessments, we found significant rater contrast effects for the Attention and Combined-Type subtypes, with evidence for a stronger rater contrast effect in the case of monozygotic pairs being obtained only in the former cases (Hudziak et al., in review).

Response to some behavior checklists, however, may be less sensitive to these biases. We have found far smaller contrast effects with the Child Behavior Checklist (CBCL), which presents symptoms alphabetically, than we did with DSM-IV interviews, which present symptoms by diagnoses (Hudziak et al. 2000).

Interviews and Questionnaires

Interviews are a social interaction and thus the data from a DSM-IV interview is affected not only by the respondent's bias (such as those described above) but also by their reaction to the interviewer. The influence of interviewer/respondent interaction on rater bias effects is unclear. The results of other twin studies, the majority of which used symptom checklist measures, also suggested that the individual symptom domains of inattention and hyperactivity (Levy et al. 1997; Sherman et al. 1997a, 1997b) are better described as existing on a continuum rather than as discrete disease entities. These same studies reported that both domains are highly heritable. Hudziak et al. (1999) used latent class analyses of DSM-IV symptoms and produced results like those of Sherman et al. (1997a). For boys, there were two separate but correlated factors, best described as Attention Problems and hyperactivity-impulsivity problems. However, the LCA results suggested that, in this sample of adolescent girls, DSM-IV symptomatology is best conceptualized in terms of three continuous problem domains that correspond to the DSM-IV conceptualization of ADHD: a domain of predominantly Attention problems, a domain of predominantly Hyperactivity-Impulsivity problems, and a domain with both Attention and Hyperactivity-Impulsivity problems.

The results revealed latent class subtypes that constitute the extremes of continuous symptom domains rather than categorical disease entities. Furthermore, the LCA raised the possibility that the DSM criteria for the Combined Type may be overly narrow (girls with 11–12 total symptoms were assigned by LCA to the severe Combined Type class, even when only 4 Hyperactivity-Impulsivity symptoms were reported) and that the criteria for predominantly Attention type may be too broad. Such data may be useful in refining future diagnostic approaches for ADHD. Because our twin sample was female, we repeated these analyses and found similar latent class structure for 7- to 17-year-old children of alcoholic parents (Neuman et al. 1999). These findings suggest that children with significant ADHD problems are not being identified when current diagnostic (DSM-IV) approaches are used. This has particularly important implications for research and assessment. Combined with the finding that each of these domains exists on a severity continuum, this suggests that a noncategorical approach to phenotype identification for those children suffering from problems with inattention and hyperactivity-impulsivity may be warranted.

Development

One obstacle to measuring phenotypes in child psychopathology is that they may change with development. In adult psychiatric genetics, the same criteria are usually applied to adults of all ages. This is based on the assumption that phenotypes such as schizophrenia are stable across adulthood. In child psychopathology, such phenotypic stability is the exception rather than the rule. Developmental psychologists have suggested that children typically pass through stages of psychological (Freud 1980), cognitive (Piaget 1954), and moral (Erickson 1963) development. As Achenbach (1982) stated, "we need to consider the developmental tasks, problems, and competencies marking successive developmental periods" (p. 1). Clearly, we must understand normal development to design developmentally sensitive phenotypic measures of child psychopathology. For example, it may not be appropriate to apply some of the criteria for ADHD to 3-year-olds (e.g., often fails to give close attention to details, makes careless mistakes in schoolwork). Similarly, the hyperactivity items of ADHD are widely acknowledged to be less prevalent in older subjects. Unless we have a strategy that can establish levels of behavior in the normal population and then relate the behavior of 3-year-olds to that of 5-, 7-, 10-, and 12-year-olds, we may misidentify true cases.

Examples of developmental change include the findings that aggressive behavior declines over the course of normal development. Conversely, we know that scores on the Delinquent Behavior Scale tend to first decrease then increase over the course of normal development (Stanger et al. 1997). Failure to control for these differences could lead to incorrect measurements of changing phenotypes. Such measurement errors may produce excessive false positives or false negatives, depending on a subject's developmental level.

In collaboration with the Missouri Twin Study, my colleagues and I analyzed CBCL data on 1,000 twin pairs. The mean age of the twins was 13.3 years, and there were equal numbers of boys and girls. We found identical heritability estimates (a^2) of 0.58 for boys and girls for Attention Problems, 0.41 for boys and 0.69 for girls for Aggressive Behavior, and 0.23 for boys and 0.44 for girls for Anxious/Depressed Behavior (Hudziak et al. 2000). These results are consistent with those reported in previous twin studies using the Achenbach-Based Approach syndromes Attention Problems, Aggressive Behavior, and Anxious/Depressed Behavior. The Anxious/Depressed Behavior a^2 varied from 0.72 in twins ages 2 and 3 to 0.50 in twins of average age 7.7, to 0.32 in twins of average age 11 (Edelbrock et al. 1995; Schmitz et al. 1995; van den Oord et al. 1995). Aggressive Behavior a^2 ranged between 0.52 and 0.69.

Although the studies used different age groups, had small samples, and were from different countries, they yielded consistent evidence of genetic influences. Attention Problems had remarkably similar heritability estimates of 0.65 to 0.66 across samples and age groups. Several questions remain to be addressed. Are there new or diminishing genetic and/or environmental effects with age? Are there differences in rates of comorbidity between the syndromes over the course of development? Finally, are there gender differences in the genetic and environmental contributions to these syndromes? Although firm conclusions cannot be drawn from these studies of twins of various ages and across different samples, the results do argue for longitudinal research to determine if the genetic influences on common behaviors change over time.

Although these data are based on self-reports and previous data are from parental reports, these data provide further evidence of developmental differences in the genetic and environmental contributions to these syndromes. Findings from this study of self-report data from 1,700 twin pairs demonstrate different levels of genetic influence across two consecutive developmental periods. The Anxious/Depressed Behavior scale had identical a^2 (0.47) and unique environmental variance (e^2, 0.53) across the adolescent period (ages 13–17) and young adulthood (ages 18–24). The same was true for Attention Problems, with an a^2 of 0.42 and an e^2 of 0.58 across developmental periods. For Aggressive Behavior, however, there were developmental effects only for females. Male adolescents had an a^2 of 0.55; for females, it was 0.20. Young adults did not differ, both having an

a^2 for Aggressive Behavior of 0.40. The cause of these gender differences is unclear; however, it is clear that more research is needed on samples of twins large enough to estimate developmental, gender-specific genetic and environmental effects at different developmental periods. Such research will expose the pathways into and out of Attention Problems, Aggressive Behavior, and Anxious/Depressed Behavior over the course of development.

Several twin studies have shown Attention Problems to be highly heritable. In fact, the heritability estimate (a^2) for Attention Problems has been remarkably similar across various samples of different age twins from numerous countries. Edelbrock et al. (1984), Hudziak et al. (2000), Schmitz et al. (1995, 1996), van den Oord et al. (1995), and van der Valk et al. (1998) all found a^2 for Attention Problems to be 0.65 or 0.66. Given the age range of subjects (3–25) and diverse informants (parents, teachers, and young adult self-reports), these studies demonstrate that the Achenbach-Based Approach provides a solid methodology to test for genetic effects. To determine if Attention Problems would meet all the Tsuang criteria, Hudziak et al. (2000) performed a family study using Attention Problems as a phenotypic marker, reporting that Attention Problems was an excellent marker for molecular genetic studies of ADHD.

Gender

Genetic studies of childhood psychopathology should allow for potential gender differences in the manifestation of genotypes. According to Hartung and Widiger (1998), of the 21 disorders usually first diagnosed in infancy, childhood, or adolescence for which sex ratios are provided, 17 have higher prevalence in boys than girls. They enumerated several sources of error that could generate or exaggerate gender differences in rates of psychopathology. Most notably, Hartung and Widiger sampled biases and biases within the diagnostic criteria, concluding that "there may not be a mental disorder for which there are not important gender differences in the manner in which the disorder is expressed" (p. 274). This seems especially true for the study of ADHD, which is three to six times more prevalent in boys than girls (Offord et al. 1987). Gaub and Carlson (1997) affirmed that research on gender differences in ADHD, with emphasis on the potential confounding effects of referral bias, comorbidity, development, diagnostic procedures, and data source, is much needed.

There are also robust gender differences in conditions that occur comorbid with ADHD. Boys are more often diagnosed with oppositional defiant disorder (ODD) and conduct disorder. Girls are more often diagnosed as having anxiety disorders (Last 1989; Lewis and Miller 1990). Prepubertal

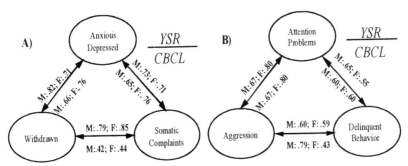

FIGURE 13-1 Across-syndrome correlations.
CBCL = Child Behavior Checklist; F = Female; M = Male; YSR = Youth Self-Report.

boys and girls have similar rates of diagnosed depression; however, during adolescence, girls show a marked increase in the rate of depression over that of boys (Brooks-Gunn and Petersen 1991; Cairns et al. 1989; Forehand et al. 1991; Rutter et al. 1986). Finally, in a genetic study, Faraone et al. (1992) reported different familial loadings and comorbidities where the probands were female rather than male.

To demonstrate how heritability estimates can be different across genders, two studies of Hudziak et al. (2000) are presented in Figures 13-2 and 13-3. The numbers above the paths are genetic correlations between the encircled syndromes for males and females from *self-report data* on 1,700 Dutch adolescent/young adult pairs (Boomsma et al., in review). The numbers below the paths represent genetic correlations between the encircled syndromes for *parental CBCL reports* on the 1,000 pairs of Missouri twins (Hudziak et al. 2000). Figure 13-2A shows the cross-syndrome correlations for the Anxious/Depressed Behavior, Somatic Complaints, and Withdrawn Behavior syndromes, which have been broadly described as "internalizing syndromes." Figure 13-2B shows the cross-syndrome correlations for the Attention Problems, Aggressive Behavior, and Delinquent Behavior syndromes, which have been broadly described as the "externalizing syndromes." For both females and males (Figure 13-2A), genetic correlations are high between Anxious/Depressed Behavior and Withdrawn Behavior as well as between Anxious/Depressed Behavior and Somatic Complaints, 0.71. This is true for self-report (Youth Self-Report [YSR]) and parental report (CBCL) data. Genetic correlations are low across Somatic Complaints and Withdrawn Behavior, 0.44 for females and 0.42 for males by self-report, yet the parent report correlations are high (0.79 for boys and 0.85 for girls). These data suggest that parents may not distinguish Withdrawn Behavior and Somatic Complaints behavior as clearly as self-reports.

On CBCL parent report data (see Figure 13-2B), findings support a strong correlation between Aggressive Behavior and Delinquent Behavior

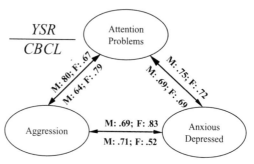

FIGURE 13-2   Across-syndrome correlations.
CBCL = Child Behavior Checklist; F = Female; M = Male; YSR = Youth Self-Report.

for males (0.79) but not for females (0.43). However, there is no difference in the genetic correlations between Aggressive Behavior and Delinquent Behavior by self-report data (0.60 for males and 0.59 for females). This illustrates the importance of considering gender, even at the level of genetic correlations between syndromes. These findings reveal gender similarities and differences that will be useful to explore in the proposed multi-informant study of twins assessed at ages 3, 7, 10, and 12.

Comorbidity

Child psychiatric geneticists who study ADHD recognize that it is often comorbid with other problems (Pliszka 1992; Semrud-Clikeman et al. 1992). A review of the literature (Hudziak and Todd 1993) reported the following rates of comorbidity: ADHD with ODD, 35%; ADHD with Conduct Disorder, 50%; ADHD with mood disorder, 15% to 75%; and ADHD with anxiety disorders, 25%. According to family studies, ADHD-ODD/Conduct Disorder signals a discrete genotype (Faraone et al. 1991), ADHD with major depression is a variable expression of the same genotype (Biederman et al. 1991a), and ADHD with anxiety disorders may be independently transmitted (Biederman et al. 1991a). Patterns of comorbidity differ if the proband is female rather than male (Faraone et al. 1991). Finally, Jensen et al. (1997) concluded their extensive review of the ADHD literature by arguing for further study of ADHD-aggressive and ADHD-anxious subtypes.

In an investigation of the bivariate genetic correlations for the comorbid CBCL syndromes Attention Problems-Aggressive Behavior (which correspond to ADHD-ODD/Conduct Disorder) and Attention Problems-Anxious/Depressed Behavior (hypothesized to be highly related to ADHD-Anxiety), we found that they are strongly intercorrelated and genetically influenced (Hudziak et al. 1998b). These data indicate shared and discrete genetic influences may contribute to comorbidity.

An important finding from the Young Adult Self-Report study is that the cross-syndrome genetic correlation between Attention Problems-Anxious/Depressed Behavior (i.e., the genetic correlation between an internalizing syndrome Anxious/Depressed Behavior and Attention Problems) was as high (0.75 for females, 0.72 for males) as the genetic correlations between Attention Problems-Aggressive Behavior (i.e., the correlation between an externalizing syndrome and Attention Problems; 0.80 for females, 0.67 for males). These results suggest that Attention Problems, Aggressive Behavior, and Anxious/Depressed Behavior in adolescent and young adult twins by self-report have both shared and independent genetic factors. Correlations for the CBCL data on the Missouri twin sample of 1,000 pairs yielded similar results with some evidence of developmental differences. The genetic correlation between Attention Problems-Aggressive Behavior was 0.69 for both males and females. The genetic correlation for Attention Problems-Anxious/Depressed Behavior was 0.69 for males and 0.83 for females and for Aggressive Behavior-Anxious/Depressed Behavior was 0.64 for males and 0.72 for females (Hudziak et al. in preparation). These findings, combined with the findings of van Gestel et al. (1997), who reported the genetic correlation for Attention Problems-Aggressive Behavior for young twins to be 1.00, indicate that Attention Problems and Aggressive Behavior may be a unitary genetic construct in very young twins (ages 2–3) and young twins (ages 6–11) may yet be affected by multiple genetic factors in older twins (ages 11–16 and 18–24).

Numerous authors have found a high degree of genetic overlap (genetic correlation) between Attention Problems and Aggressive Behavior. In a Belgian sample of 760 twins, ages 6–16, van Gestel et al. (1997) reported that, when their sample was split into a younger group (ages 6–11) and an older group (ages 12–16), the following a^2 emerged—the a^2 for Attention Problems was 0.57 for the young and 0.87 for the old, and the a^2 for Aggressive Behavior was 0.75 for both groups. In bivariate analysis, the genetic correlations between Attention Problems-Aggressive Behavior for the young group was 1.00 (consistent with Attention Problems-Aggressive Behavior being a unitary genetic construct) and 0.74 for the older group (consistent with Attention Problems and Aggressive Behavior having both independent and shared genetic risks). Hudziak et al. (1998b) found the genetic correlation between Attention Problems and Aggressive Behavior of 0.69 for males and females. This work correlates with the findings of Silberg et al. (1994), who used the Rutter Questionnaire to define the Attention Problems and Aggressive Behavior domains. These two studies collapsed large age ranges of children in their analysis (ages 6–11 and 12–16), yet found consistent results supporting high genetic correlations between Attention Problems and Aggressive Behavior. Boomsma (personal communication, June 1999) found a genetic correlation between Attention

Problems and Aggressive Behavior of 0.74 for a large sample of 3-year-old Dutch twins.

In a twin study using the YSR and Young Adult Self-Report, Boomsma and Hudziak (in preparation) reported that the genetic correlation between Attention Problems and Aggressive Behavior was 0.67 for both males and females. The phenotypic and environmental correlations were between 0.45 and 0.55, reflecting the role of environment in the expression of these traits. These studies are consistent with the results of bivariate genetic analysis of the relations between DSM-IV ADHD and ODD/Conduct Disorder as measured by a 10-item telephone survey conducted by Nadder et al. (1998). In their study of 900 twin pairs, ages 7–13, they reported that the genetic correlation between ADHD and ODD/Conduct Disorder was 50%, replicating previous findings of a common genetic factor influencing the comorbidity between symptoms of ADHD and ODD/Conduct Disorder.

Similar to Attention Problems and Aggressive Behavior, Attention Problems and Anxious-Depressed Behavior also share high genetic correlations. Hudziak et al. (1998b) reported genetic correlations on CBCL data between Attention Problems and Anxious-Depressed Behavior to be 0.69 for males and 0.83 for females. In a related analysis, Hudziak et al. (in review) reported genetic correlations between Attention Problems and Anxious-Depressed Behavior for males (0.72) and for females (0.75). These data argue for further studies of the comorbid Attention Problems–Anxious-Depressed Behavior subtype. In summary, Anxious-Depressed Behavior has been shown to be heritable, to correlate with DSM anxiety and depressive disorders, and to co-occur with Attention Problems and Aggressive Behavior in twin studies.

FUTURE APPROACHES

Developmentally informed studies that follow the same sample of children, prospectively, and that take into account multiple informants and use multiple measures will likely improve our ability to identify highly heritable and refined phenotypes. These phenotypes can then be used in association, linkage, and quantitative trait loci studies, and perhaps, to identify genetic and environmental risk factors for common child psychiatric conditions.

CONCLUSION

The new medical genetics and its molecular, population, and statistical techniques offers child psychiatry a cadre of tools that will improve our ability to diagnose and treat children who suffer from emotional and behavioral disorders. To take advantage of these remarkable advances, child psychiatry must enhance the likelihood that scientific expeditions into gene discovery are informed by a taxonomy that meets the criteria of a genetic nosology. Our taxonomy should meet the rules of Tsuang et al. (1993) and should be sensitive to the confounds of development, gender, informant bias, instrument bias, categories and continua, and comorbidity. Once tested, molecular genetics will likely then inform subsequent iterations of this taxonomy. Future studies should use molecular genetic findings to improve our ability to define phenotypes, which could then be used in subsequent molecular genetic studies to iteratively refine our taxonomy. As we refine our taxonomic approach, we may have more success identifying genetic and environmental risks for ADHD. Such an approach will most likely result in a taxonomy that is truly both phenotypic and genotypic. For example, in the future, children with ADHD may well be described as ADHD-Dopamine 4 Receptor Gene (7), ADHD-Dopamine Transporter Gene (10), and ADHD-Dopamine 3 Receptor Gene. If the power of the new medical genetics is achieved, treatments may vary by genotype. These interventions, in concert with behavioral and cognitive behavioral therapies, may lead to improved outcomes for children and adults with ADHD. Given the remarkable techniques that are currently available and others that will almost certainly follow, child psychiatry serves to greatly benefit from the new medical genetics.

REFERENCES

Achenbach TM: Developmental Psychopathology, 2nd Edition. New York, Wiley, 1982

Achenbach TM: Taxonomy and comorbidity of conduct problems: evidence from empirically based approaches. Special issue: toward a developmental perspective on Conduct Disorder. Dev Psychopathol 5(1–2):51–64, 1993

American Psychiatric Association: Diagnostic and Statistical Manual of Mental Disorders, Third Edition, Revised (DSM-III-R). Washington, DC, American Psychiatric Association, 1987

American Psychiatric Association: Diagnostic and Statistical Manual of Mental Disorders, Fourth Edition (DSM-IV). Washington, DC, American Psychiatric Association, 1994

Biederman J, Faraone SV, Keenan K, et al: Evidence of familial association between attention deficit disorder and major affective disorders. Arch Gen Psychiatry 48(7):633–642, 1991a

Biederman J, Faraone SV, Keenan K, et al: Familial association between attention deficit disorder and anxiety disorders. Am J Psychiatry 148(2):251–256, 1991b

Brooks-Gunn J, Petersen AC: Studying the emergence of depression and depressive symptoms during adolescence. Special issue: the emergence of depressive symptoms during adolescence. J Youth Adolesc 20(2):115–119, 1991

Cairns RB, Cairns BD, Neckerman HJ, et al: Growth and aggression, I: childhood to early adolescence. Dev Psychol 25(2):320–330, 1989

Eaves LJ, Silberg JL, Maes HH, et al: Genetics and developmental psychopathology, 2: the main effects of genes and environment on behavioral problems in the Virginia Twin Study of Adolescent Behavioral Development. J Child Psychol Psychiatry 38(8):965–980, 1997

Edelbrock C, Costello AJ, Kessler MD: Empirical corroboration of attention deficit disorder. J Am Acad Child Psychiatry 23(3):285–290, 1984

Edelbrock C, Rende R, Plomin R, et al: A twin study of competence and problem behavior in childhood and early adolescence. J Child Psychol Psychiatry 36(5):775–785, 1995

Erickson E: Childhood and Society. New York, Norton, 1963

Faraone SV, Biederman J, Chen WJ, et al: Segregation analysis of attention deficit hyperactivity disorder. Psychiatr Genet 2(4):257–275, 1992

Faraone SV, Biederman J, Keenan K, et al: Separation of DSM-III attention deficit disorder and Conduct Disorder: evidence from a family genetic study of American child psychiatric patients. Psychol Med 21(1):109–121, 1991

Forehand R, Neighbors B, Wierson M: The transition of adolescence: the role of gender and stress in problem behavior and competence. J Child Psychol Psychiatry 32(6):929–937, 1991

Freud A: Child analysis as the study of mental growth, in The Course of Life: Psychoanalytic Contributions Toward Understanding Personality Development. Edited by Greenspan SI, Pollack GH. Madison, CT, International Universities Press, 1980

Gaub M, Carlson CL: Gender differences in ADHD: a meta-analysis and critical review. J Am Acad Child Adolesc Psychiatry 36(8):1036–1045, 1997

Goodman R, Stevenson J: A twin study of hyperactivity, I: an examination of hyperactivity scores and categories derived from Rutter teacher and parent questionnaires. J Child Psychol Psychiatry 30(5):671–689, 1989a

Goodman R, Stevenson J: A twin study of hyperactivity, II: the aetiological role of genes, family relationships and perinatal adversity. J Child Psychol Psychiatry 30(5):691–709, 1989b

Hartung CM, Widiger TA: Gender differences in the diagnosis of mental disorders: conclusions and controversies of the DSM-IV. Psychol Bull 123(3):260–278, 1998

Hudziak JJ, Todd R: Familial subtyping of attention deficit hyperactivity disorder. Curr Opin Psychiatry 6:489–493, 1993

Hudziak JJ, Heath AC, Madden PAF, et al: Latent class and factor analysis of DSM-IV ADHD: a twin study of female adolescents. J Am Acad Child Adolesc Psychiatry 37(8):848–857, 1998a

Hudziak JJ, Heath AC, Rudiger LP, et al: A twin study of CBCL syndromes: the genetics of comorbidity. Data presented at the American Academy of Child and Adolescent Psychiatry, Anaheim, CA, Scientific Proceedings, 1998b, pp 127–128

Hudziak JJ, Wadsworth ME, Heath AC, et al: Latent class analysis of Child Behavior Checklist Attention Problems. J Am Acad Child Adolesc Psychiatry 38:8, 1999

Hudziak J, Rudiger L, Neale M, et al: A twin study of inattentive, aggressive, and anxious/depressed behaviors. J Acad Child Adolesc Psychiatry 39(4):469–476, 2000

Jensen PS, Martin D, Cantwell DP: Comorbidity in ADHD: implications for research, practice, and DSM-V. J Am Acad Child Adolesc Psychiatry 36(8):1065–79, 1997

Jensen PS, Shervette RE, Xenakis SN, et al: Anxiety and depressive disorders in attention deficit disorder with hyperactivity: new findings. Am J Psychiatry 150(8):1203–1209, 1993

Knowles ES, Byers B: Reliability shifts in measurement reactivity: driven by content engagement or self-engagement? J Pers Soc Psychol 70(5):1080–1090, 1996

Langer EJ, Imber L: The role of mindlessness in the perception of deviance. J Pers Soc Psychol 39:360–367, 1980

Last CG: Anxiety Disorders. Edited by Ollendick TH, Hersen, M. New York, Plenum Press, 1989

Levy F, Hay DA, McStephen M, et al: Attention-deficit hyperactivity disorder: a category or a continuum? Genetic analysis of a large-scale twin study. J Am Acad Child Adolesc Psychiatry 36(6):737–744, 1997

Lewis M, Miller SM: Handbook of Developmental Psychopathology. New York, Plenum Press, 1990

Nadder TS, Silberg JL, Eaves LJ, et al: Genetic effects on ADHD symptomatology in 7- to 13-year-old twins: results from a telephone survey. Behav Genet 28(2):83–99, 1998

Neale MC, Cardon LR, North Atlantic Treaty Organization, Scientific Affairs Division: Methodology for Genetic Studies of Twins and Families. Boston, MA, Kluwer Academic Publishers, 1992

Neale MC, Walters EE, Eaves LJ, et al: Multivariate genetic analysis of twin-family data on fears: Mx models. Behav Genet 24(2):119–139, 1994

Neuman RJ, Todd RD, Heath AC, et al: The evaluation of ADHD typology in three contrasting samples: a latent class approach. J Am Acad Child Adolesc Psychiatry 38:25–33, 1999

Offord DR, Boyle MH, Szatmari P, et al: Ontario Child Health Study, II: six-month prevalence of disorder and rates of service utilization. Arch Gen Psychiatry 44(9): 832–836, 1987

Piaget J: The Construction of Reality in the Child. New York, Basic Books, 1954

Pliszka SR: Comorbidity of attention-deficit hyperactivity disorder and overanxious disorder. J Am Acad Child Adolesc Psychiatry 31(2):197–203, 1992

Rutter M: Child psychiatric disorder: measures, causal mechanisms, and interventions (comment). Arch Gen Psychiatry 54(9):785–789, 1997

Rutter M, Izard CE, Read PB: Depression in young people: developmental and clinical perspectives. New York, Guilford Press, 1986

Schmitz S, Fulker DW, Mrazek DA: Problem behavior in early and middle childhood: an initial behavior genetic analysis. J Child Psychol Psychiatry 36(8):1443–1458, 1995

Schmitz S, Saudino KJ, Plomin R, et al: Genetic and environmental influences on temperament in middle childhood: analyses of teacher and tester ratings. Child Dev 67(2):409–422, 1996

Schwarz N: Self-reports: how the questions shape the answers. Am Psychol 54(2):93–105, 1999

Semrud-Clikeman M, Biederman J, Sprich-Buckmister S, et al.: Comorbidity between ADHD and learning disability: a review and report in a clinically referred sample. J Am Acad Child Adolesc Psychiatry 31(3):439–448, 1992

Sherman DK, Iacono WG, McGue MK: Attention-deficit hyperactivity disorder dimensions: a twin study of inattention and impulsivity-hyperactivity. J Am Acad Child Adolesc Psychiatry 36(6):745–753, 1997a

Sherman DK, McGue MK, Iacono WG: Twin concordance for attention deficit hyperactivity disorder: a comparison of teachers' and mothers' reports. Am J Psychiatry 154(4):532–535, 1997b

Silberg JL, Erickson MT, Meyer JM, et al: The application of structural equation modeling to maternal ratings of twins' behavioral and emotional problems. Special section: structural equation modeling in clinical research. J Consult Clin Psychol 62(3):510–521, 1994

Stanger C, Achenbach TM, Verhulst FC: Accelerated longitudinal comparisons of aggressive versus delinquent syndromes. Dev Psychopathol 9(1):43–58, 1997

State M, Lombroso P, Pauls D, et al: The genetics of childhood psychiatric disorders: a decade of progress. J Am Acad Child Adolesc Psychiatry 39(8):946–962, 2000

Thapar A, Hervas A, McGuffin P: Childhood hyperactivity scores are highly heritable and show sibling competition effects: twin study evidence. Behav Genet 25(6):537–544, 1995

Tsuang MT, Faraone SV, Lyons MJ: Identification of the phenotype in psychiatric genetics. Special issue: genetic epidemiology of psychiatric disorders. Eur Arch Psychiatry Clin Neurosci 243(3–4):131–142, 1993

van den Oord EJCG, Koot HM, Boomsma DI, et al: A twin-singleton comparison of problem behaviour in 2–3-year-olds. J Child Psychol Psychiatry 36(3):449–458, 1995

van der Valk JC, Verhulst FC, Stroet TM, et al: Quantitative genetic analysis of Internalising and Externalising problems in a large sample of 3-year-old twins. Twin Res 1(1):25–33, 1998

van Gestel S, Danckaerts M, Verhelle B, et al: Genetic and Environmental Influence on the Covariation Between Hyperactivity, Delinquency, and Aggression Scores on the CBCL. Toronto, 1997

Verhulst FC, van der Ende J, Ferdinand RF, et al: The prevalence of DSM-III-R diagnoses in a national sample of Dutch adolescents. Arch Gen Psychiatry 54:329–336, 1997

14

Defining Genetically Meaningful Classes of Psychopathology

Stephen V. Faraone, Ph.D.

Since the 1980s, a revolution has taken place in the statistical and molecular genetic techniques of gene finding. The discovery of disease genes has created a new age of molecular medicine and drug development. To date, gene finding has been most successful for well-defined disorders with simple modes of inheritance. In contrast, although genetic epidemiological studies overwhelmingly implicate genes in the etiology of mental disorders, researchers in psychiatric genetics have yet to clone a gene that predisposes to psychopathology. Although future breakthroughs in psychiatric genetics may come from large-scale linkage studies, it is possible that they will also require an improved "psychiatric genetic nosology." This chapter discusses methods for defining genetically meaningful phenotypes and illustrates these methods with data from studies of schizophrenia and attention-deficit hyperactivity disorder (ADHD).

The new millennium of research into the genetic basis of psychopathology offers new vistas for research and new hopes for treatment. For many psychiatric disorders, there is a sturdy foundation of genetic epidemiological data showing that genes influence susceptibility to illness (Faraone

This work was supported in part by National Institute of Mental Health Grants R01MH57934, R01HD37694, and R01HD37999 to Dr. Faraone.

et al. 1999a). Upon this foundation, molecular and statistical genetic technologies promise to build an enduring structure that will house solutions to many questions of etiology, pathophysiology, diagnosis, and treatment. However, geneticists and statisticians will not succeed without continued advances by psychiatric epidemiologists and clinical investigators. Indeed, the failure to replicate linkage findings in schizophrenia (Tsuang et al. 1999) and mood disorders (Tsuang and Faraone 1990) suggests that methods that are routinely successful for simple Mendelian illnesses will not fare well with psychiatric disorders.

Clearly, the clinical and epidemiological features of psychiatric disorders raise many questions for genetic studies (Diehl and Kendler 1989; Elston and Wilson 1990; Gershon 1990; Green 1990; Matthysse 1990; Merikangas et al. 1989; Morton 1990; Ott 1990a, 1990b; Risch 1990a; Suarez et al. 1990; Weeks et al. 1990). This chapter focuses on one of these questions: how do we define genetically meaningful classes of psychopathology?

PSYCHIATRIC GENETIC NOSOLOGY

Kendler (1990) introduced the term "scientific nosology" to describe nosological systems used to formulate and test hypotheses. Tsuang et al. (1993) used the term "psychiatric genetic nosology" to describe to a scientific nosology created from psychiatric genetic data. Ideally, a psychiatric genetic nosology would classify patients into categories that correspond to distinct genetic entities. Such a nosology need not be useful for clinicians, nor should it be viewed as a replacement for DSM-IV (American Psychiatric Association 1994) or ICD-10 (World Health Organization 1992). Instead, a psychiatric genetic nosology seeks to define disorders in a manner that is most useful for genetic studies.

A psychiatric genetic nosology must address the problem of diagnostic accuracy (i.e., the degree to which a diagnosis correctly classifies people with and without a putative genetic illness). When dealing with a categorical diagnosis, the fundamental types of inaccuracy are false positives and false negatives. *False positives* refer to subjects who are incorrectly diagnosed as being ill. *False negatives* refer to subjects incorrectly diagnosed as being well. A genetic perspective on diagnostic accuracy must address two issues: etiological heterogeneity and reduced penetrance.

When several genetic and nongenetic factors can independently cause disease, people with and without the disease might be accurately discriminated against; however, it may be difficult to discriminate against subtypes. From a measurement perspective, etiological heterogeneity creates a second class of false positives, that is, subjects who are correctly classified as having an illness but incorrectly classified as having a genetic subform of the illness. For example, some patients diagnosed as having Alzheimer's disease do not have the diagnosis confirmed on autopsy; these patients correspond to the traditional definition of a false positive. Among all patients who have the disease at autopsy, all will be true positives for the illness but false positives for all but one subform (e.g., a patient with a chromosome 21 mutation would be a false positive in studies of the chromosome 14 variant). Thus, there are two types of false positives and both make it difficult to detect genes for etiologically heterogeneous disorders. Thus, false positives diminish statistical power and reduce evidence for linkage (Ott 1991a).

Reduced penetrance means that the pathogenic genotype does not always produce illness. Thus, low penetrance is an issue of diagnostic accuracy because it indicates that some gene carriers will be misclassified because they do not express the illness. Low penetrance seems to be the rule rather than the exception for psychiatric disorders. For example, when one member of a monozygotic twin pair has schizophrenia (Gottesman and Shields 1982), bipolar disorder (Tsuang and Faraone 1990), major depression (Tsuang and Faraone 1990), ADHD (Faraone and Doyle 2000), or panic disorder (Crowe 1990), the probability of the co-twin being ill is well below 100%. Although this could indicate etiological heterogeneity (some cases may not be genetic), it also suggests a role for reduced penetrance. Reduced penetrance creates a second type of false negative, that is, subjects who carry the gene but are correctly diagnosed as not having the disease.

METHODS FOR DEALING WITH DIAGNOSTIC INACCURACY

Many methods have been put forth to solve the problem of misclassification in genetic studies. Purely statistical methods have been in use for some time. These include linkage analysis with affected members (Weeks and Lange 1988) or model parameterizations that include reduced penetrance and etiological heterogeneity (Ott 1991a). These either ignore or model misclassification, but, in contrast to clinical and epidemiological approaches, they do not directly address issues of nosology.

Some methods deal with the nosological issues of genetic studies by starting with known categories and reorganizing them to improve the informativeness of family data. When the genotype that causes a psychiatric disorder has variable manifestations, we say that the genotype has variable expressivity. Whereas *penetrance* describes the probability that the genotype will be manifested as a specific illness, *expressivity* indicates that the occurrence of the clinical phenotype is not an all-or-none phenomenon; that is, there may be quantitative gradations of being affected or qualitative differences in gene expression. The variable expressivity of genotypes for psychiatric disorders may produce a "spectrum" of both clinical and non-clinical phenomena (Faraone et al. 1999a).

There are many examples of variable expressivity in psychiatry. The schizophrenia genotype may produce schizoaffective disorder, schizotypal personality, and atypical psychotic disorders (Tsuang et al. 1999, 2000). The biological relatives of bipolar patients are at high risk for major depressive and bipolar II disorders (Tsuang and Faraone 1990). The familial predisposition for panic disorder appears to express itself in childhood anxiety disorders and laboratory measures of inhibited behavior (Rosenbaum et al. 2000). Obsessive-compulsive disorder (OCD) and chronic tics are alternate manifestations of Tourette syndrome (TS; Pauls et al. 1986). The genotype for ADHD may express itself as mood, conduct, or antisocial personality disorders (Faraone and Doyle 2000).

In addition to clinical expression of psychopathology, we must also consider the value of neurobiological phenotypes. These have been studies extensively in families of patients with schizophrenia. These studies have found several neurobiological abnormalities that appear to reflect the actions of schizophrenia genes in nonschizophrenic people. Examples are smooth pursuit eye movement dysfunction (Arolt et al. 1996; Iacono et al. 1992), the auditory evoked potentials (Blackwood et al. 1991b; Freedman et al. 1997), visual sustained attention (Erlenmeyer-Kimling et al. 1991; Neuchterlein and Dawson 1984), neuropsychological impairment (Faraone et al. 1999b), and neuroimaging assessed brain abnormalities (Seidman et al. 1997).

Keefe et al. (1991) defined three types of phenotypic indicators. *Diagnostic indicators* are deficits that are more common among individuals with a disease compared with control subjects. These are not secondary to external factors such as medication use and are not state dependent. They may not be useful for genetic studies because they could be sequelae of the nongenetic factors that cause disease expression. *Spectrum indicators* meet the criteria for diagnostic indicators but are also found in subjects with disorders that are believed to be genetically related to the disease. Thus, spectrum indicators may reflect the effects of the genotype that cause the disease. Because they are found in nondiseased relatives, they cannot be attributed to secondary effects of the disease. *Phenotypic indicators* are diagnostic indicators that show evidence for genetic transmission, and they are found among relatives of diseased probands (even if the relatives do not have the disease). Phenotypic indicators may be useful for linkage analyses because they identify affected family members who cannot be classified as affected by psychiatric measures alone.

However, we must use phenotypic indicators with caution. When many are available for a single disease, problems may arise. For example, we already know of several clinical and neurobiological phenotypic indicators for schizophrenia. When a linkage study collects several of these, it becomes possible to test for linkage using many different definitions of who is and is not affected. This increases the risk that a positive linkage finding will be due to chance alone. There are statistical solutions to this problem (Goldin 1990; Green 1990; Ott 1990a), but each of these is accompanied by some loss in statistical power.

Thus, phenotypic indicators must be used judiciously. One way to do this is to define a diagnostic hierarchy prior to linkage analyses (Merikangas et al. 1989; Weeks et al. 1990). The top level of the hierarchy includes the core definition of the illness. Subsequent levels use increasingly broader definitions. For example, at its top level, a schizophrenia linkage study could include schizophrenia and schizoaffective disorder, depressed. At the second level, psychotic disorder not otherwise specified and schizotypal personality disorder could be added. A third level could add individuals who exhibit oculomotor, attentional, or neuropsychological impairments. The first level minimizes the likelihood of false-positive diagnoses. As lower levels are included, the sensitivity will be increased but there is an associated decrement in specificity (i.e., the false-positive rate increases).

There is a second problem with phenotypic indicators: they may be useless for genetic studies. Phenotypic indicators are helpful because they decrease the false-negative rate (i.e., they increase penetrance). However, this decrease in the false-negative rate is usually accompanied by an increase in the false-positive rate (i.e., the phenotypic indicators are usually more prevalent among control subjects than the disease under study). For example, the rate of oculomotor dysfunction among relatives of schizophrenic patients ranges from 14% to 50% (Blackwood et al. 1991a; Clementz et al. 1992; Holzman et al. 1974, 1977, 1984; Iacono et al. 1992). Because this is greater than the 10% rate of schizophrenia and related psychoses (Gottesman and Shields 1982), oculomotor dysfunction decreases the false-negative rate. However, this ignores a key point: although rates of oculomotor impairment are statistically greater among relatives of patients with schizophrenia compared with control subjects, the rate among control subjects is not negligible (2% to 8%; Blackwood et al. 1991a; Clementz et al. 1992; Holzman et al. 1974, 1977, 1984; Iacono et al. 1992). This suggests that the use of oculomotor measures as a phenotypic indicator may increase false positives.

The work of Risch (1990b, 1990c) suggests a simple method for assessing whether the tradeoff between false negatives and false positives makes a phenotypic indicator more or less useful. He showed that the power of a linkage study is directly related to the ratio of two prevalences: the prevalence among relatives of ill probands and the prevalence in the general population. The greater the ratio, the more power. Thus, one way to increase the statistical power of linkage analysis is to define a phenotype that is highly prevalent among relatives of ill probands but rare in the general population. It follows that a phenotype indicator will be most useful if it increases the prevalence ratio. If it maintains the same ratio, it may be useful by increasing the number of pedigrees informative for linkage analysis. For example, families with two or more cases of schizophrenia are rare; their ascertainment is a difficult, time-consuming, and expensive process (Chen et al. 1992; Pulver and Bale 1989). Many more families would be informative if we use phenotypic indicators to designate affection.

Faraone et al. (1995a) examined 30 studies of several putative indicators of the schizophrenia genotype: schizotypal and paranoid personality disorders and traits, eye-tracking dysfunction, attentional impairment, neurological signs/neuropsychological impairment, allusive thinking, and auditory evoked potentials. The 30 studies provided a total of 42 data points because some studies computed rates of impairment based on different thresholds of impairment or different definitions of the outcome variable.

As discussed earlier, Risch (1990c) suggested that defining disease status in a manner that increased the prevalence ratio would increase the power of linkage analyses. For a schizophrenia phenotype that comprises schizophrenia and other psychoses, the risk to offspring and siblings is approximately 10% and the population prevalence is 1% (Tsuang et al. 1999). Thus, for offspring and siblings, the prevalence ratio for the psychosis phenotype is approximately 10. The use of a spectrum phenotype for schizophrenia would modify this prevalence ratio as follows. First, when using the spectrum phenotype, the rate of being "affected" among relatives will equal the 10% rate of psychotic disorders plus the rate of the spectrum phenotype among the nonpsychotic relatives of patients with schizophrenia (this is called sensitivity [SN]). Second, the estimated rate of affected individuals in the population will be equal to the 1% rate of schizophrenia and related psychotic disorders in the population, plus the rate with which the spectrum phenotype is observed among the control group (in this context, this latter rate is the false-positive rate [FP]). Then, the prevalence ratio, P_s, for the spectrum phenotype will be as follows:

$$P_s = \frac{10 + (SN \times 90)}{1 + (FP \times 99)} \qquad (1)$$

For a spectrum indicator to be useful, it must, at the very least, lead to a prevalence ratio, P_s, that equals 10—the prevalence ratio of the psychosis phenotype. After substituting $P_s = 10$ into equation (1), we derived the following:

$$SN = 11 \times FP \tag{2}$$

Equation (2) shows that, for the psychosis plus spectrum phenotype to retain the same prevalence ratio as the psychosis phenotype, the sensitivity of the spectrum phenotype must be 11 times greater than its false-positive rate.

Figure 14-1 shows the distribution of prevalence ratios computed by Faraone et al. (1995a). Notably, of the 42 spectrum phenotypes analyzed, only 3 had prevalence ratios exceeding 10 and only 1, an attention composite score from the New York High Risk Study (Cornblatt et al. 1989), was markedly greater (30). Since this review was published, Faraone et al. (1995b) computed a prevalence ratio of 36 neuropsychological composite score. This work clearly shows that, although a putative spectrum phenotype may differentiate relatives of schizophrenic patients from control subjects, it may not be useful for linkage analyses.

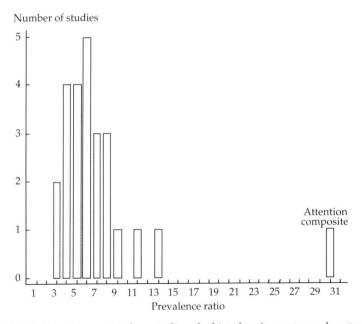

FIGURE 14-1   Prevalence ratios from studies of schizophrenia-spectrum phenotypes.

DEALING WITH ETIOLOGICAL HETEROGENEITY

The discussion in the previous section shows how Risch's model provides a useful framework for assessing the utility of phenotypic indicators that result from the variable expression of psychiatric genotypes. His method is also useful for the assessment of phenotypic variability due to etiological heterogeneity. But, before his method can be applied, we need some means of defining genetically meaningful subtypes of disorder.

Pauls (1986) suggested that data from family studies could answer this question. In his studies of TS and OCD he posited the following: If OCD is a variable expression of TS, then the relatives of probands with TS should have elevated rates of OCD, regardless of whether the proband also had OCD. If OCD is only found among relatives of those probands having both TS and OCD, then there are two possibilities. TS and OCD may be independently transmitted disorders, or TS with OCD may be a genetic subtype of TS. If the latter is the case, then TS and OCD should not be independently transmitted in the families of probands with both disorders. That is, in these families, relatives with TS should have higher rates of OCD than relatives without TS.

In some ways, the approach advocated by Pauls et al. (1986) is an essential phase of analysis because so many psychiatric disorders occur comorbidly with other disorders (Boyd et al. 1984). For example, ADHD is associated with conduct disorder, major depression, anxiety disorders, and learning disabilities (Biederman et al. 1991a). A series of family genetic analyses suggests that the presence of conduct disorder signals a discrete subtype of the disorder and major depression is a variable expression of the disorder, but anxiety and learning disabilities appear to be independently transmitted from ADHD (Biederman et al. 1991b; Faraone and Biederman 1997; Faraone et al. 1993, 1997, 1998b). Such findings provide useful guides for genetic studies of ADHD; that is, they stratify probands based on the presence of conduct disorder and they count major depression—but not anxiety or learning disabilities—as a spectrum indicator.

FINE-TUNING THE FALSE-POSITIVE AND FALSE-NEGATIVE RATES

Tsuang et al. (1993) proposed a simple method of fine-tuning the false-positive and false-negative rates of diagnosis. For psychiatric disorders, measurement error creates a difficult problem because we have no gold standard to define who is and is not affected (Faraone and Tsuang 1994). Thus, the two traditional indices of diagnostic accuracy—sensitivity (the probability that an affected subject is diagnosed as affected) and specificity (the probability that an unaffected subject is diagnosed as unaffected)—are difficult, if not impossible, to compute.

Fortunately, as an extensive literature in epidemiology and biostatistics shows, the sensitivity and specificity of a diagnostic procedure change in predictable ways when we combine the results of multiple diagnostic procedures in a systematic fashion (Gastwirth 1987; Lau 1989, 1991; McClish and Quade 1985; Politser 1982; Quade et al. 1980). These methods use simple diagnostic rules, which work even when the underlying sensitivity and specificity of the procedures are unknown. These diagnostic rules are as follows:

1. Use the diagnosis of one diagnostician as the final diagnosis.
2. Obtain two diagnoses and record the final diagnosis as ill only if *both* diagnosticians diagnose the subject as ill.
3. Obtain two diagnoses and record the final diagnosis as ill if *either* diagnostician diagnoses the subject as ill.
4. Use three diagnosticians.

The final diagnosis is recorded as ill if a *majority* of the three conclude that the subject is ill.

To determine the potential utility of these rules, Tsuang et al. (1993) simulated their sensitivities and specificities. They found that, compared with a single diagnosis, using two diagnosticians (rule 2) increased specificity and decreased sensitivity. They found the reverse trend for rule 3, which decreased specificity and increased sensitivity. To improve both sensitivity and specificity required more than two diagnosticians and the use of rule 4.

Notably, the "best" diagnostic rule depends on the sensitivity and specificity of a single diagnostician. If these are poor, then the more complex rules cannot create a phenotype definition that will be useful for linkage analyses. In contrast, when either or both are large, then it becomes possible to construct a very accurate phenotype definition. For example, when the sensitivity is 0.6 and the specificity 0.9 (for a single diagnostician), the use of three diagnosticians achieves a specificity of 0.96 (which is nearly perfect).

The choice of a diagnostic rule cannot be divorced from its goals. Because false positives can mask the presence of linkage (Greenberg 1992; Ott 1991a), a psychiatric genetic nosology should seek maximum specificity while maintaining reasonable levels of sensitivity. This goal would favor rule 2 because this can dramatically increase specificity. The utility of any of these rules can, of course, be tested using Risch's prevalence ratios as described earlier.

DEFINING NEW PHENOTYPES

In the previous sections, the use of predefined categories for genetic studies was discussed. Another approach tries to define new phenotypes that maximally correspond to the genetic component of psychiatric illnesses. Although the official diagnostic nomenclature used by clinicians and most researchers treats diagnoses as discrete entities, measurement approaches in the psychological literature (Achenbach 1992; Lord and Novick 1968) focus on dimensional traits that can take on a range of values. A measure of "caseness" provides a compromise. It is a dimensional measure of the degree to which we believe that a subject is truly ill.

The idea of caseness fits well with the realities of diagnosis. Some patients clearly have a disorder; others certainly do not. Many more fall between the extremes of diagnostic clarity. It is sensible to associate each of these uncertain cases with an index of caseness that expresses the probability that they truly have the disorder. Although such an index would not necessarily deal with the genetic level of diagnostic error, it should facilitate genetic analyses to the degree that it corresponds to the true (but unobservable) illness status of the subject.

Ott (1991b) showed how linkage analyses could use measures of caseness by assigning subjects weights indicating the probability that they are affected. These weights can be subjective probability judgments made by diagnosticians or predictions made by mathematical models of disease expression. In a linkage analysis algorithm, these weights can be used to determine the penetrance of each genotype for diagnoses made with varying degrees of certainty.

We can use caseness measures to summarize the multiple sources of diagnostic and neurobiological data that bear on the definition of psychiatric phenotypes. Instead of conducting several analyses that test linkage to a hierarchy of conditions, each condition can be assigned a weight that indicates the probability that a subject with the condition has the genotype. For example, in a schizophrenia linkage study a subject with schizophrenia might be given a weight of 1, a subject with schizotypal personality and oculomotor dysfunction a weight of 0.8, and a subject with either schizotypal personality or oculomotor dysfunction a weight of 0.6.

An index of caseness can also be derived from stability data (Rice et al. 1987, 1992). Rice et al. (1987, 1992) reasoned that stable diagnoses are more likely to reflect a true underlying illness than other diagnoses. To define an index of caseness based on stability, they used clinical measures from patients with mood disorder diagnoses (e.g., number of symptoms or episodes) to predict who would and would not report a lifetime history of the disorder 6 years later. The result of this procedure is a logistic regression equation that uses the clinical measures to compute the probability that a case will be stable, which is an index of caseness that could be used in a genetic study.

We have shown the potential for stability to be an effective measure of caseness in studies of ADHD (Biederman et al. 1996a; Faraone et al. 2000). ADHD is known to have a strong genetic component (Faraone and Doyle 2000), yet its low prevalence ratio (about 5.0) suggests that using the clinical diagnosis to find genes will be difficult.

Faraone et al. (2000) proposed that stable or persistent ADHD might be a useful subtype of ADHD for genetic studies. They reasoned that cases that remit before adolescence might have a smaller genetic component to the disorder than persistent cases. One of their studies examined 140 boys with ADHD and 120 boys without ADHD at a baseline assessment and completed a prospective 4-year follow-up study. By mid-adolescence, 85% of boys with ADHD continued to have ADHD, and 15% remitted. The prevalence of ADHD among parents was 16.3% for the persistent ADHD probands and 10.8% for the remitted ADHD probands. For siblings, the respective prevalences were 24.4% and 4.6%. Thus, these data suggest that children with persistent ADHD have a more familial form of ADHD than those whose ADHD remits by adolescence (Biederman et al. 1996b).

Biederman et al. (1995) also demonstrated the increased familiality of persistent ADHD in two retrospective studies. In a pilot study, they showed that children of clinically referred parents with childhood-onset ADHD were at high risk for meeting diagnostic criteria for ADHD: 84% of the adults with ADHD who had children had at least one child with ADHD and 52% had two or more children with ADHD. The 57% rate of ADHD among children of adults with ADHD was much higher than the more modest 15% risk for ADHD in siblings of referred children with this disorder (Faraone et al. 1992). These findings were consistent with a prior study by Manshadi et al. (1983) that studied the siblings of 22 alcoholic adult psychiatric patients who met DSM-III (American Psychiatric Association 1980) criteria for attention-deficit disorder (ADD), residual type. The authors compared these patients with 20 patients matched for age and comorbid psychiatric diagnoses. Forty-one percent of the siblings of the adult probands with ADD were diagnosed with ADHD, compared with 0% of the comparison siblings without ADHD.

In another retrospective study, Biederman et al. (1998) compared adolescents with ADHD that retrospectively reported childhood-onset ADHD with children with ADHD. They found that the relatives of adolescent probands had higher rates of ADHD compared with the relatives of child probands. Thus, a prospective study of children and retrospective studies

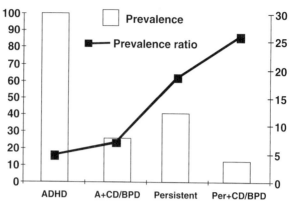

FIGURE 14-2   Prevalence and prevalence ratios for four ADHD phenotypes. ADHD = attention-deficit/hyperactivity disorder; A + CD/BPD = ADHD with conduct or bipolar disorder; Persistent = Persistent ADHD, Per + CD/BPD = Persistent ADHD with conduct or bipolar disorder.

of adolescents and adults all suggested that, when ADHD persists into adolescence and adulthood, it is highly familial.

To determine if the persistent ADHD phenotype would be useful for genetic studies, Faraone et al. (2000) computed Risch's prevalence ratio for persistent ADHD and compared that with prevalence ratios for all ADHD cases and for ADHD subgroups defined by psychiatric comorbidity with conduct or bipolar disorders. This latter group was chosen because prior work suggests that children with ADHD who have either of these disorders were a distinct familial type (Faraone et al. 1998a).

The results of this work are given in Figure 14-2, which shows both the sample prevalence (the vertical bars) and the prevalence ratios (squares connected by lines) for the four ADHD phenotypes. By definition, the prevalence of ADHD among probands was 100%. The prevalence ratio for the ADHD families was about 5.0. ADHD with conduct or bipolar disorder (A + CD/BPD) was seen in 22% of the probands. Their families yielded a slightly higher prevalence ratio. The prevalence of persistent ADHD among probands was about 13%; the prevalence ratio was much higher at about 20%. When probands were selected for being both persistent and having conduct or bipolar disorder (Per + CD/BPD), the prevalence was less than 5% but the prevalence ratio was much higher (25%).

These results show that the persistence of ADHD selects families that are at very high risk for ADHD. As Figure 14-2 shows, the increases in Risch's prevalence ratio are substantial, which suggest that families selected through persistent ADHD probands will have more statistical power for linkage analysis compared with families selected without regard to persistence.

Although the persistent conduct disorder/bipolar disorder phenotype led to the greatest prevalence ratio, that phenotype was relatively rare, affecting less than 5% of the probands. In contrast, about 13% met criteria for a persistent syndrome and these probands still had a substantial recurrence risk among both siblings and parents. These considerations suggest that persistent ADHD probands would be a suitable and practical phenotype to use for pedigree selection. Of course, investigators having access to very large ADHD populations or to those enriched with persistent conduct disorder/bipolar disorder cases would do better to focus on this highly familial phenotype.

CONCLUSION

Psychiatric genetics is at a crossroads. Genetic epidemiological studies show without a doubt that genes play a major role in the etiology of most forms of psychopathology. Yet, although molecular genetic studies have implicated many broad chromosomal regions, they have not yet found a specific gene for any psychiatric disorder. The ambiguity of these molecular genetic studies may be clarified by the collection of very large samples, now under way at several centers around the world. However, it is also possible that standard molecular genetic methods will require novel psychiatric phenotypes (i.e., genetically meaningful classes of psychopathology).

This chapter illustrates that there are several approaches to creating genetically meaningful classes of psychopathology. These approaches should be useful for creating the genetic nosology proposed by Tsuang et al. (1993). Their potential utility in the search for genes has been illustrated by two studies of schizophrenia. Furthermore, the approaches showed that the use of eye tracking (Arolt et al. 1996) and P50-evoked potential measures (Freedman et al. 1997) as phenotypes suggested linkage where the clinical diagnosis did not. Whether they will ultimately facilitate the identification of genes for psychopathology awaits future research.

REFERENCES

Achenbach TM: Manual for the Child Behavior Checklist/2–3 and 1992 Profile. Burlington, VT, University of Vermont, Department of Psychiatry, 1992

American Psychiatric Association: Diagnostic and Statistical Manual of Mental Disorders, 3rd Edition (DSM-III). Washington, DC, American Psychiatric Association, 1980

American Psychiatric Association: Diagnostic and Statistical Manual of Mental Disorders, 4th Edition (DSM-IV). Washington, DC, American Psychiatric Association, 1994

Arolt V, Lencer R, Achim N, et al: Eye tracking dysfunction is a putative phenotypic susceptibility marker of schizophrenia and maps to a locus on chromosome 6p in families with multiple occurrence of the disease. Am J Med Genet 67:564–579, 1996

Biederman J, Newcorn J, Sprich SE: Comorbidity of attention deficit hyperactivity disorder with conduct, depressive, anxiety, and other disorders. Am J Psychiatry 148:564–577, 1991a

Biederman J, Faraone SV, Keenan K, et al: Familial association between attention deficit disorder and anxiety disorders. Am J Psychiatry 148:251–256, 1991b

Biederman J, Faraone SV, Mick E, et al: High risk for attention deficit hyperactivity disorder among children of parents with childhood onset of the disorder: a pilot study. Am J Psychiatry 152:431–435, 1995

Biederman J, Faraone S, Milberger S, et al: Predictors of persistence and remission of ADHD: results for a three-year prospective follow-up study of ADHD children. J Am Acad Child Adolesc Psychiatry 35:343–351, 1996a

Biederman J, Faraone SV, Milberger S, et al: Predictors of persistence and remission of ADHD: results from a four-year prospective follow-up study of ADHD children. J Am Acad Child Adolesc Psychiatry 35:343–351, 1996b

Biederman J, Faraone SV, Taylor A, et al: Diagnostic continuity between child and adolescent ADHD: findings from a longitudinal clinical sample. J Am Acad Child Adolesc Psychiatry 37:305–313, 1998

Blackwood DHR, St. Clair D, Muir WJ, et al: Auditory P300 and eye tracking dysfunction in schizophrenic pedigrees. Arch Gen Psychiatry 49:899–909, 1991a

Blackwood D, St. Clair D, Muir W: DNA markers and biological vulnerability markers in families multiply affected with schizophrenia. Eur Arch Psychiatry Neurol Sci 240:191–196, 1991b

Boyd JH, Burke JD, Gruenberg E, et al: Exclusion criteria of DSM-III: a study of co-occurrence of hierarchy-free syndromes. Arch Gen Psychiatry 41:983–989, 1984

Chen WJ, Faraone SV, Tsuang MT: Linkage studies of schizophrenia: a simulation study of statistical power. Genet Epidemiol 9:123–139, 1992

Clementz BA, Grove WM, Iacono WG, et al: Smooth-pursuit eye movement dysfunction and liability for schizophrenia: implications for genetic modeling. J Abnorm Psychol 101:117–129, 1992

Cornblatt B, Winters L, Erlenmeyer-Kimling L: Attentional markers of schizophrenia: evidence from the New York High-Risk Study, in Schizophrenia: Scientific Progress. Edited by Schulz SC, Tamminga CA. New York, Oxford University Press, 1989, pp 83–92

Crowe RR: Panic disorder: genetic considerations. J Psychiatr Res 24:129–134, 1990

Diehl SR, Kendler KS: Strategies for linkage studies of schizophrenia: pedigrees, DNA markers, and statistical analyses. Schizophr Bull 15:403–419, 1989

Elston RC, Wilson AF: Genetic linkage and complex diseases: a comment. Genet Epidemiol 7:17–19, 1990

Erlenmeyer-Kimling L, Rock D, Squires-Wheeler E, et al: Early life precursors of psychiatric outcomes in adulthood in subjects at risk for schizophrenia or affective disorders. Psychiatr Res 39:239–256, 1991

Faraone SV, Biederman J: Do attention deficit hyperactivity disorder and major depression share familial risk factors? J Nerv Ment Dis 185:533–541, 1997

Faraone SV, Doyle A: Genetic influences on attention deficit hyperactivity disorder. Curr Psychiatry Rep 2:143–146, 2000

Faraone SV, Tsuang MT: Measuring diagnostic accuracy in the absence of a gold standard. Am J Psychiatry 151:650–657, 1994

Faraone S, Biederman J, Chen WJ, et al: Segregation analysis of attention deficit hyperactivity disorder: evidence for single gene transmission. Psychiatr Genet 2:257–275, 1992

Faraone SV, Biederman J, Krifcher B, et al: Evidence for independent transmission in families for Attention Deficit Hyperactivity Disorder (ADHD) and learning disability: results from a family genetic study of ADHD. Am J Psychiatry 150:891–895, 1993

Faraone SV, Kremen WS, Lyons MJ, et al: Diagnostic accuracy and linkage analysis: how useful are schizophrenia spectrum phenotypes? Am J Psychiatry 152:1286–1290, 1995a

Faraone SV, Seidman LJ, Kremen WS, et al: Neuropsychological functioning among the nonpsychotic relatives of schizophrenic patients: a diagnostic efficiency analysis. J Abnorm Psychol 104:286–304, 1995b

Faraone SV, Biederman J, Garcia Jetton J, et al: Attention deficit disorder and conduct disorder: longitudinal evidence for a familial subtype. Psychol Med 27:291–300, 1997

Faraone SV, Biederman J, Mennin D, et al: Bipolar and antisocial disorders among relatives of ADHD children: parsing familial subtypes of illness. Am J Med Genet 81:108–116, 1998a

Faraone SV, Biederman J, Mennin D, et al: Familial subtypes of attention deficit hyperactivity disorder: a four year follow-up study of children from antisocial-ADHD families. J Child Psychol Psychiatry 39:1045–1053, 1998b

Faraone SV, Tsuang D, Tsuang MT: Genetics of Mental Disorders: A Guide for Students, Clinicians, and Researchers. New York, Guilford, 1999a

Faraone SV, Seidman LJ, Kremen WS, et al: Neuropsychological functioning among the nonpsychotic relatives of schizophrenic patients: a four-year follow-up study. J Abnorm Psychol 108:176–181, 1999b

Faraone SV, Biederman J, Monuteaux M: Toward guidelines for pedigree selection in genetic studies of attention deficit hyperactivity disorder. Genet Epidemiol 18:1–16, 2000

Freedman R, Coon H, Myles-Worsley M, et al: Linkage of a neurophysiological deficit in schizophrenia to a chromosome 15 locus. Proc Natl Acad Sci U S A 94:587–592, 1997

Gastwirth JL: The statistical precision of medical screening procedures: application to polygraph and AIDS antibodies test data. Stat Sci 2:213–238, 1987

Gershon ES: Genetic linkage and complex diseases: a comment. Genet Epidemiol 7:21–23, 1990

Goldin LR: The increase in type I error rates in linkage studies when multiple analyses are carried out on the same data: a simulation study (abstract). Am J Hum Genet 47:A180, 1990

Gottesman II, Shields J: Schizophrenia: The Epigenetic Puzzle. Cambridge, MA, Cambridge University Press, 1982

Green P: Genetic linkage and complex diseases: a comment. Genet Epidemiol 7:25–27, 1990

Greenberg DA: There is more than one way to collect data for linkage analysis: what a study of epilepsy can tell us about linkage strategy for psychiatric disease. Arch Gen Psychiatry 49:745–750, 1992

Holzman PS, Proctor LR, Levy DL, et al: Eye-tracking dysfunctions in schizophrenic patients and their relatives. Arch Gen Psychiat 31:143–151, 1974

Holzman PS, Kringlen E, Levy DL, et al: Abnormal-pursuit eye movements in schizophrenia: evidence for a genetic indicator. Arch Gen Psychiatry 34:802–805, 1977

Holzman PS, Solomon CM, Levin S, et al: Pursuit eye movement dysfunction in schizophrenic patients and their relatives. Arch Gen Psychiatry 44:1140–1141, 1984

Iacono WG, Moreau M, Beiser M, et al: Smooth-pursuit eye tracking in first-episode psychotic patients and their relatives. J Abnorm Psychol 101:104–116, 1992

Keefe RSE, Silverman JM, Siever LJ, et al: Refining phenotype characterization in genetic linkage studies of schizophrenia. Soc Biol 38:197–218, 1991

Kendler KS: Toward a scientific psychiatric nosology: strengths and limitations. Arch Gen Psychiatry 47:969–973, 1990

Lau T-S: On repeated screening tests. Biometrics 45:891–898, 1989

Lau T-S: On dependent repeated screening tests. Biometrics 47:77–86, 1991

Lord FM, Novick MR: Statistical Theories of Mental Test Scores. Reading, MA, Addison-Wesley, 1968

Manshadi M, Lippmann S, O'Daniel R, et al: Alcohol abuse and attention deficit disorder. J Clin Psychiatry 44:379–380, 1983

Matthysse S: Genetic linkage and complex diseases: a comment. Genet Epidemiol 7:29–31, 1990

McClish D, Quade D: Improving estimates of prevalence by repeated testing. Biometrics 41:81–89, 1985

Merikangas KR, Spence A, Kupfer DJ: Linkage studies of bipolar disorder: methodologic and analytic issues. Report of MacArthur Foundation workshop on linkage and clinical features in affective disorders. Arch Gen Psychiatry 46:1137–1141, 1989

Morton NE: Genetic linkage and complex diseases: a comment. Genet Epidemiol 7:33–34, 1990

Neuchterlein KH, Dawson ME: Information processing and attentional functioning in the developmental course of schizophrenic disorders. Schizophr Bull 10:160–203, 1984

Ott J: Genetic linkage and complex diseases: a comment. Genet Epidemiol 7:35–36, 1990a

Ott J: Invited editorial: cutting a Gordian knot in the linkage analysis of complex human traits. Am J Hum Genet 46:219–221, 1990b

Ott J: Analysis of Human Genetic Linkage. Baltimore, MD, The Johns Hopkins University Press, 1991a

Ott J: Genetic linkage analysis under uncertain disease definition, in Banbury Report 33: Genetics and Biology of Alcoholism. Edited by Cloninger CR, Begleiter H. Cold Springs Harbor, NY, Cold Spring Harbor Laboratory Press, 1991b, pp 327–331

Pauls DL, Towbin KE, Leckman JF, et al: Gilles de la Tourette's syndrome and obsessive-compulsive disorder: evidence supporting a genetic relationship. Arch Gen Psychiatry 43:1180–1182, 1986

Politser P: Reliability, decision rules, and the value of repeated tests. Med Decis Making 2:47–69, 1982

Pulver AE, Bale SJ: Availability of schizophrenic patients and their families for genetic linkage studies: findings from the Maryland epidemiology sample. Genet Epidemiol 6:671–680, 1989

Quade D, Lachenbruch PA, Whaley FS: Effects of misclassifications on statistical inferences in epidemiology. Am J Epidemiol 111:503–515, 1980

Rice JP, Endicott J, Knesevich MA, et al: The estimation of diagnostic sensitivity using stability data: an application to major depressive disorder. J Psychiatr Res 21:337–345, 1987

Rice JP, Rochberg N, Endicott J, et al: Stability of psychiatric diagnoses: an application to the affective disorders. Arch Gen Psychiatry 49:824–830, 1992

Risch N: Genetic linkage and complex diseases, with special reference to psychiatric disorders. Genet Epidemiol 7:3–7, 1990a

Risch N: Linkage strategies for genetically complex traits, I: multilocus models. Am J Hum Genet 46:222–228, 1990b

Risch N: Linkage strategies for genetically complex traits, II: the power of affected relative pairs. Am J Hum Genet 46:229–241, 1990c

Rosenbaum JF, Biederman J, Kagan J, et al: A controlled study of behavioral inhibition in children of parents with panic disorder and depression. Am J Psychiatry 157:2002–2010, 2000

Seidman LJ, Faraone SV, Goldstein JM, et al: Reduced subcortical brain volumes in nonpsychotic siblings of schizophrenic patients: a pilot MRI Study. Am J Med Genet 74:507–514, 1997

Suarez BK, Reich T, Rice JP, et al: Genetic linkage and complex diseases: a comment. Genet Epidemiol 7:37–40, 1990

Tsuang MT, Faraone SV: The Genetics of Mood Disorders. Baltimore, MD, The Johns Hopkins University Press, 1990

Tsuang MT, Faraone SV, Lyons MJ: Identification of the phenotype in psychiatric genetics. Eur Arch Psychiatry Neurol Sci 243:131–142, 1993

Tsuang MT, Stone WS, Faraone SV: Schizophrenia: a review of genetic studies. Harv Rev Psychiatry 7:185–207, 1999

Tsuang MT, Stone WS, Faraone SV: Towards reformulating the diagnosis of schizophrenia. Am J Psychiatry 147:1041–1050, 2000

Weeks DE, Brzustowicz L, Squires-Wheeler E, et al: Report of a workshop on genetic linkage studies in schizophrenia. Schizophr Bull 16:673–686, 1990

Weeks DE, Lange K: The affected-pedigree-member method of linkage analysis. Am J Hum Genet 42:315–326, 1988

World Health Organization: International Statistical Classification of Diseases and Health Problems, 10th Revision. Geneva, Switzerland, World Health Organization, 1992

15

Schizotaxia and the Prevention of Schizophrenia

Ming T. Tsuang, M.D., Ph.D.

Although substantial progress has been achieved in both the diagnosis and treatment of schizophrenia, a full understanding of its origins and pathogenic mechanisms remains elusive. Understanding the development of schizophrenia is critical for developing new treatment strategies, in part because early interventions (i.e., secondary prevention) are associated with better treatment outcomes. There is thus a growing emphasis on the accurate diagnosis of schizophrenia as soon as symptoms of psychosis are evident. Conceptually, of course, the most effective treatment would involve the prevention of psychosis altogether (i.e., primary prevention).

Progress toward this goal remains in its infancy, however, in part because we are only just learning to identify what the genetic liability to schizophrenia looks like *before* the onset of the prodromal period, which is when symptoms are often first noticed. This chapter reviews progress in this

Preparation of this chapter was supported in part by the National Institute of Mental Health Grants 1R01MH4187901, 5UO1MH4631802 and 1R37MH4351801 to Dr. Ming T. Tsuang; the Veterans Administration's Medical Research, Health Services Research and Development and Cooperative Studies Programs; and by a NARSAD Distinguished Investigator Award to Dr. Tsuang.

area by focusing on *schizotaxia*, a clinically meaningful condition that may reflect the liability for schizophrenia. The discussion of schizotaxia begins by considering implications of the longstanding diagnosis of schizophrenia as a discrete, psychotic illness, whose clinical symptoms are unrelated to their underlying etiological mechanisms. The concept of schizotaxia is then presented as an alternative formulation of schizophrenic illness that contains an important clinical implication: the possibility of developing treatment strategies for the primary prevention of schizophrenia. Finally, our initial attempts to identify and treat schizotaxia are reviewed.

LIMITATIONS OF THE CURRENT VIEW OF SCHIZOPHRENIA

It is now generally agreed that stringent, narrow diagnostic criteria for schizophrenia and other mental disorders were needed in the 1970s and 1980s to improve the reliability of clinical diagnoses (e.g., Tsuang et al. 2000). Periodic revisions of the major classificatory systems have refined diagnoses further, increased their reliability, facilitated the task of differential diagnosis, and provided the basis for empirical methods to determine which symptoms most appropriately characterized specific disorders. The reliability of diagnosis provided by recent DSMs and ICDs has also benefited research to the extent that the clinical characteristics of samples are more standardized across studies, which makes them easier to replicate. Moreover, the use of stringent diagnostic criteria laid the groundwork for studies to assess the validity of the concept.

Despite the many advances of DSM-III (American Psychiatric Association 1980) and its successors, we may still consider how the classification of schizophrenia could be improved further. This is not intended as a criticism of our progress thus far, but instead reflects the need to modify our conceptual and classificatory schemes as new information becomes available. In this context, at least three limitations of the current diagnostic criteria may be addressed, including its emphasis on psychosis, its definition of schizophrenia as a discrete category, and its dissociation of symptoms from their etiology. Each of these limitations leads to the same issues: can the validity of the diagnostic criteria for schizophrenia be increased while its reliability is retained? More specifically, is the current classification of schizophrenia the most accurate reflection available of the genetic and environmental risk factors that produce it? Most important, from a practical point of view, would alternative conceptions of schizophrenia promote the development of novel treatment strategies? These issues are considered next.

Psychosis and the Definition of Schizophrenia

Psychosis has long been the *sine qua non* for schizophrenia (Tsuang et al. 2000), but is it really a specific component of the disorder or more of a nonspecific indicator of severe mental illness? The latter view has support because psychosis is not specific to schizophrenia or to other psychiatric conditions. It occurs, for example, in many neurological disorders (e.g., Alzheimer's disease, Huntington's disease, schizophrenia-like psychosis of epilepsy, vascular dementia, traumatic brain injury) and can be caused by a range of toxic substances or impaired metabolic states. Even Schneiderian first-rank symptoms, which played a prominent role in defining the nature of psychotic symptoms in modern diagnostic systems, are not specific for schizophrenia (Peralta and Cuesta 1998). In fact, measures of psychosis per se do not always differentiate schizophrenia clearly from other forms of psychopathology (Bell et al. 1998; Peralta et al. 1997; Ratakonda et al. 1998) and, at some psychotic symptoms, often overlap between different psychotic disorders (Serretti et al. 1996).

Interestingly, a number of molecular genetic studies that did not detect linkage to schizophrenia on the basis of DSM diagnoses showed stronger evidence for linkage when the phenotype was broadened to include additional psychotic disorders (e.g., Maziade et al. [1997] at chromosome 6p and Wildenauer et al. [1996] at chromosome 18p). Moreover, different psychotic disorders may share common genetic elements or chromosomal loci (Tsuang et al. 1999a). Schizoaffective disorder, for example, might belong to an affective disorder spectrum as well as to a schizophrenia disorder spectrum (Bertelsen and Gottesman 1995; Wildenauer et al. 1999). Consistent with this view, schizoaffective disorder occurs in families with either schizophrenia or affective disorders. More generally, both schizophrenia and affective disorders occur at elevated rates in families with either disorder (e.g., Maier et al. 1993).

Similarities between psychotic symptoms in different disorders may reflect inherent pathophysiological effects of psychosis. In support of this view, 1) clinical outcomes of schizophrenia improve when treatment is obtained early in the illness (Wyatt 1995), 2) some patients with schizophrenia show neurobiological abnormalities (Knoll et al. 1998), and 3) common abnormalities, such as in GABA-ergic neurotransmission, may occur across psychotic conditions (Keverne 1999).

What are the implications of similarities in psychotic symptoms? Crow (1990, 1991) proposed a continuum of psychosis that crosses diagnostic boundaries. In so doing, he accepted the view that prototypical entities corresponded to schizophrenia and affective illness but rejected the idea that they had distinct etiologies. Instead, he proposed that psychotic disorders shared a common genetic basis. Although support for this view is weak, Crow's view of psychosis is intriguing. If, in fact, psychosis has an etiology apart from other core symptoms of schizophrenia, then our longstanding diagnostic focus on psychosis in schizophrenia could be a mistake. In the hunt for the causes of schizophrenia, psychosis could be a red herring, or a "fever" of severe mental illness (i.e., a serious but nonspecific indicator of an underlying disorder). Because psychotic states may impair functioning in a relatively global manner and may have adverse neuropathological effects of their own, their net effect may be to emphasize superficial similarities between such disorders, while obscuring more subtle, but defining, differences between them.

DSM-IV Schizophrenia as a Discrete Category

Like other disorders, DSM-IV (American Psychiatric Association 1994) defines schizophrenia as a discrete category rather than a quantitative dimension. An implicit implication of this classification is that schizophrenia begins with the onset of its symptoms as listed in DSM-IV. Before that time, the disorder cannot be recognized validly; that is, if the criteria for other disorders also are not met, then individuals cannot receive any psychiatric diagnoses. To a significant degree, the cut point for making the decision is whether psychotic symptoms are present.

In general, a reliance on discrete categories raises potential problems for cases that share symptoms of multiple disorders because they may lead to artificial boundary categories and elevated rates of comorbidity (Frances et al. 1991). Certainly, dimensional models of psychopathology have conceptual and pragmatic limitations as well (Frances et al. 1991; Millon 1991), but the question remains as to whether a dimensional model describes the biological nature of schizophrenia more accurately than a categorical one. Is it more valid? Certainly, a dimensional view of schizophrenia is more consistent (than a categorical one) with polygenic models of inheritance, which is the model that provides the best account of the familial transmission of schizophrenia (Gottesman 1991; Tsuang et al. 1999a). Polygenic models assume that multiple genes combine with one another and with environmental factors to cause schizophrenia. Because multiple genes and environmental risk factors are involved, it is possible for people to have low, moderate, or high "doses" of risk factors that predispose to schizophrenia. People with very high doses are at high risk for schizophrenia; those with moderate doses may have related conditions such as schizotypal personality disorder, negative symptoms, neuropsychological impairment, or other neurobiological manifestations of the predisposition to schizophrenia (Faraone et al. 1995a). It thus seems clear that a dimensional model describes the range of schizophrenic illness better than a categorical one.

In fact, a partial foundation for a dimensional view of the biological/clinical manifestations of the vulnerability to schizophrenia already exists in the body of research about *schizotaxia*, a term introduced by Meehl (1962) to describe the unexpressed genetic predisposition to schizophrenia. Meehl suggested that individuals with schizotaxia would develop either schizotypy or schizophrenia, depending on the protection or liability afforded by environmental circumstances, although he later proposed that schizotaxia did not always progress into either of these more overt conditions (Meehl 1989). Given current data showing that, in addition to genes, environmental events (e.g., obstetric complications, viruses) augment susceptibility to schizophrenia, Faraone et al. (2000) proposed that we use the term *schizotaxia* to indicate the premorbid, neurobiological substrate of schizophrenia.

Decades of research show schizotaxia to be a clinically meaningful condition, with distinct psychiatric and neurobiological features, such as negative symptoms, neuropsychological impairment, impaired eye tracking, and structural brain abnormalities (Faraone et al. 2001). Schizotaxia is a broader construct than schizophrenia. Our empirical studies suggest that the basic symptoms of schizotaxia occur in 20%–50% of first-degree relatives of patients with schizophrenia (Faraone et al. 1995a, 1995b), compared with about 10% of relatives who will become psychotic and less than 10% who will develop schizotypal personality disorder (Battaglia and Torgersen 1996). These figures suggest that schizotaxia does not lead inevitably to schizotypal personality or to schizophrenia but in most cases is a long-term condition. This raises the issue of what type of etiological model accounts best for a long-term biological vulnerability (schizotaxia) that, in some cases, leads to psychosis (schizophrenia) and, in others, does not.

Diagnostic Criteria for Schizophrenia Ignore Its Etiology and Pathophysiology

DSM-III (and later DSM editions) explicitly dissociated diagnostic criteria from speculation about etiology to avoid incorporating theories of etiology that were not subjected to empirical tests. At this point, however, DSM-III's rejection of theoretical speculation about etiology should not lead us to reject empirical facts about etiology as being relevant to diagnosis or conceptualization. Moreover, such a view risks a continuing disconnection of treatment from etiology. Since the introduction of antipsychotic medications, pharmacologic treatments have focused on alleviating the most acute, florid symptoms of schizophrenia (i.e., those related to psychosis). Although several newer antipsychotic medications also alleviate selected negative symptoms and cognitive deficits, treatment remains symptomatic. It is not aimed at correcting specific causes of the disorder, nor is it aimed at preventing its onset.

It is uncommon to think of psychosis as a nonspecific end state of schizophrenia, but this is reasonable in light of evidence that schizophrenia's pathophysiology begins long before the first psychotic episode. Such data are consistent with neurodevelopmental models of schizophrenia that posit adverse genetic and environmental interactions (e.g., Weinberger 1994, 1995; Woods 1998). These events create a neurodevelopmental syndrome that, as studies of relatives of schizophrenic patients have shown, is characterized by neuropsychological, psychophysiological, and neurobiological abnormalities (Faraone et al. 2001). For reasons that are still unknown, this syndrome sometimes leads to psychosis and sometimes does not. Notably, these indicators of the syndrome are more proximal to schizophrenia's initial causes than is psychosis.

Clinical Implications

Taken together, the evidence described earlier supports the idea that schizophrenic disorder begins before the onset of psychosis and expresses itself biologically in characteristic ways. One way to integrate these findings is to conceptualize its manifestations (e.g., biological abnormalities, biological relatedness to a family member with schizophrenia, selected neuropsychological deficits, history of obstetric complications) as risk factors that vary along dimensions of severity for schizophrenia. Schizotaxia describes this premorbid, yet clinically significant, neurodevelopmental condition. Psychosis, in contrast, represents more of a relatively less specific consequence of schizophrenic disease than does schizotaxia. If this view is correct, then the clinical significance of schizotaxia is related to both its (putative) status as a discrete condition and its status as a risk factor for schizophrenia.

The emphasis on prepsychotic *and* preprodromal aspects of schizophrenic disorder (i.e., schizotaxia) has potentially significant implications for the treatment of schizophrenia. For one, the identification of a premorbid condition, especially one that is itself clinically significant, will facilitate the development of early intervention strategies. This leads to the issue of whether psychosis can be avoided. Can schizophrenic illness be treated before psychosis is added to it? Most researchers have approached the issue of primary prevention by focusing on prodromal symptoms as indicators of an impending psychotic disorder, but such symptoms are often nonspecific (Larsen and Opjordsmoen 1996; McGorry et al. 1995). Under these circumstances, and taking account of the clinical and psychosocial risks of labeling people as preschizophrenic, the application of primary prevention programs seems premature in the absence of clear clinical symptoms.

Among the steps that will make prevention efforts more feasible for nonpsychotic individuals are identifying the population at risk and developing a rationale for treatment. The study of schizotaxia may help to achieve this goal (Faraone et al., in press). Given this hypothesis, what are the next steps that must be taken to design a strategy aimed at preventing schizophrenia? Clearly, the validity of schizotaxia as a predictor of subsequent schizophrenia must be firmly established. As Robins and Guze (1970) pointed out, it is crucial to establish both the concurrent and predictive validity of putative syndromes. Does the classification of schizotaxia predict neuropsychological, neuroimaging, or biological findings that are consistent with what is known about the neurobiology of schizophrenia? As reviewed elsewhere, a growing body of literature suggests that the answer is "yes" (Faraone et al., in press). Abnormalities found among relatives of patients with schizophrenia include eye-tracking dysfunction, allusive thinking, neurological signs, characteristic auditory evoked potentials, neuroimaging-assessed brain abnormalities, and neuropsychological impairment. Moreover, children at risk for schizophrenia show features of schizotaxia that predict subsequent schizophrenia and related disorders (Faraone et al. 2001).

Although schizotaxic features cannot yet be used to select preschizophrenic children for primary prevention protocols, current knowledge about schizotaxia suggests a method for evaluating medications that may someday be useful for the prevention of schizophrenia. This method, which we call the "schizotaxia treatment protocol," is straightforward: select a sample of schizotaxic first-degree relatives of schizophrenic patients and, using standard randomized clinical trial methodology, determine if a putative preventative treatment modifies the features of schizotaxia in a brief period of trial. Presumably, any medicine that mitigates the features of schizotaxia will be a reasonable candidate for a primary prevention trial when such trials are possible. The use of the schizotaxia treatment protocol assumes that the syndrome of schizotaxia observed among first-degree relatives of patients with schizophrenia shares etiological and pathophysiological pathways with preschizophrenic people. If this assumption is true, then any medication that targets these pathways to mitigate schizotaxic features also may work to reduce the likelihood of the onset of psychosis. This assumption is reasonable because 1) first-degree relatives of patients with schizophrenia are at high risk for carrying schizophrenia susceptibility genes (Gottesman 1991), and 2) the features of schizotaxia observed among these relatives are similar to the features of schizotaxia seen in children who eventually become schizophrenic (Faraone et al. 2001).

A major advantage of the schizotaxia treatment protocol is that it can avoid some of the ethical issues raised by primary prevention studies of schizophrenia. Prevention studies will label children and adolescents as potential future schizophrenics, which opens up the possibility of stigmatization and psychological harm to the subjects and their families. It is also possible that medications chosen for prevention trials may pose greater risks to children and adolescents than adults. That would preclude their use in the absence of a solid rationale for efficacy. However, because schizotaxia can be defined in the adult relatives of schizophrenic patients, using an acute schizotaxia trial for putative preventative medicines will not require studies of children or adolescents.

If successful treatments are developed and tested, and the syndrome of schizotaxia is validated, then treatments at earlier ages may be considered. For example, if a brief schizotaxia treatment trial in adults is successful, one might consider an acute trial for adolescents. If an adolescent trial were to be successful, then we might consider a trial to prevent psychosis (assuming that the target, preschizophrenic population could be accurately defined).

One of the difficulties with implementing the schizotaxia treatment protocol is the lack of a consensual definition of schizotaxia. Although we can make many measurements of schizotaxic features (e.g., neuropsychological symptoms, negative symptoms, social functioning), the field has yet to agree on how these measures should be combined to create a schizotaxic category. Tsuang et al. (1999b) described a working definition of schizotaxia based on a set of specific criteria for the purpose of developing a treatment protocol. In this initial approach, schizotaxia was diagnosed in people who had at least one relative with schizophrenia, an estimated IQ of 70 or higher, no lifetime history of psychotic disorders, no substance abuse diagnosis within 6 months of the evaluation, no head injury with documented loss of consciousness exceeding 5 minutes (or subsequent cognitive deficits), no history of neurological disease or damage, no medical condition with significant cognitive sequelae, and no history of electroconvulsive treatment.

Clinically, potential subjects had at least moderate levels of negative symptoms, defined as six items rated 3 or higher on the Scale for the Assessment of Negative Symptoms (SANS); moderate or greater deficits (defined as approximately two or more standard deviations below appropriate norms) in at least one of three cognitive domains (attention, long-term verbal memory, and executive functions); and deficits at least one standard deviation below normal in a second cognitive domain (see Tsuang et al. [1999b] for lists of specific tests and measures on tests used to meet the neuropsychological criteria).

Our decision to require moderate deficits in different domains ensured that our initial treatment attempts would include only adults with demonstrable clinical and neuropsychological difficulties. This was important to demonstrate both the clinically meaningful nature of schizotaxia and to make the risk/benefit assessment of treatment more favorable. Our first application of the schizotaxia treatment protocol (Tsuang et al. 1999b) used low doses of risperidone, a novel antipsychotic medication that reduces positive and some negative symptoms in schizophrenia (Marder and Meibach 1994; Rossi et al. 1997; Tamminga 1997). Notably, it also improves cognitive functions in schizophrenia, especially in attention (Green et al. 1997; Rossi et al. 1997; Stip 1996), but possibly in verbal long-term memory (Stip 1996) and executive functions (Rossi et al. 1997) as well.

After the entrance criteria were met, subjects received low doses (starting at 0.25 mg and reaching maximum doses of 2.0 mg) of risperidone for 6 weeks. During that period, they were evaluated weekly for side effects and for clinical and neuropsychological effects of treatment. After 6 weeks, most clinical and neuropsychological tests were repeated. We reported on the effects of treatment in our first four cases (Tsuang et al. 1999b) and have since completed two additional cases. Five out of six cases thus far showed marked improvements in a demanding test of auditory attention, and the same five out of six cases showed reduced negative symptoms after 6 weeks. Side effects, when they occurred, were mild to modest in severity. No one requested the discontinuation of treatment, but in some cases the doses were lowered to reduce discomfort. The individual who did not improve with treatment had a lower IQ than the other subjects (75, compared with a range of 92–111 in the other subjects), which suggests the possibility that a higher level of overall cognitive ability was necessary to benefit from the 6-week course of treatment.

CONCLUSION

Initial application of the schizotaxia treatment protocol is encouraging, although the preliminary nature of these findings needs to be underscored. Use of risperidone or other medications to treat schizotaxia is not recommended until larger, controlled studies determine that the treatment implications of these pilot findings are correct.

Despite this caveat, however, findings suggest the feasibility of developing treatment strategies for adult schizotaxia. It is clear that this process is only starting. Perhaps the most important tasks for the near future, in addition to the need for more methodologically rigorous replications, is the validation of schizotaxia as a syndrome. To accomplish this task, it will be useful to change our conceptualization of schizophrenia somewhat from the historical view of a discrete, categorical entity whose diagnosis depended on the clinical symptoms of psychosis. Instead, a more fruitful approach may be to incorporate a dimensional, neurodevelopmental perspective on schizophrenia that includes neurobiological and neuropsychological measures occurring prior to the development of psychosis (schizotaxia). As the validity of schizotaxia becomes established, the risk (for subsequent psychosis) provided by its component features will become measurable. As an initial step in this process, we have begun to compare subjects who met our criteria for schizotaxia with subjects who did not, on independent measures of clinical function (i.e., the Physical Anhedonia Scale, Social Adjustment Scale, Quality of Life Scale, Symptom Checklist-90-R, the Global Assessment of Functioning Scale). These analyses are in progress. Eventually, our knowledge base will provide the foundation for strategies aimed at the prevention of schizophrenia.

REFERENCES

American Psychiatric Association: Diagnostic and Statistical Manual of Mental Disorders, 3rd Edition (DSM-III). Washington, DC, American Psychiatric Association, 1980

American Psychiatric Association: Diagnostic and Statistical Manual of Mental Disorders, 4th Edition (DSM-IV). Washington, DC, American Psychiatric Association, 1994

Battaglia M, Torgersen S: Schizotypal disorder: at the crossroads of genetics and nosology. Acta Psychiatr Scand 94:303–310, 1996

Bell RC, Dudgeon P, McGorry PD, et al: The dimensionality of schizophrenia concepts in first-episode psychosis. Acta Psychiatr Scand 97:334–342, 1998

Bertelsen A, Gottesman II: Schizoaffective psychoses: genetical clues to classification. Am J Med Genet 60:7–11, 1995

Crow TJ: The continuum of psychosis and its genetic origins: the sixty-fifth Maudsley lecture. Br J Psychiatry 156:788–797, 1990

Crow TJ: The search for the psychosis gene. Br J Psychiatry 158:611–614, 1991

Faraone SV, Kremen WS, Lyons MJ, et al: Diagnostic accuracy and linkage analysis: how useful are schizophrenia spectrum phenotypes? Am J Psychiatry 152:1286–1290, 1995a

Faraone SV, Seidman LJ, Kremen WS, et al: Neuropsychological functioning among the nonpsychotic relatives of schizophrenic patients: a diagnostic efficiency analysis. J Abnorm Psychol 104:286–304, 1995b

Faraone SV, Green AI, Seidman LJ, et al: "Schizotaxia": clinical implications and new directions for research. Schizophr Bull 27:1–18, 2001

Frances AJ, First MB, Widiger TA, et al: An A to Z guide to DSM-IV conundrums. J Abnorm Psychol 100:407–412, 1991

Gottesman II: Schizophrenia Genesis: The Origin of Madness. New York, Freeman, 1991

Green MF, Marshall BDJ, Wirshing WC, et al: Does risperidone improve verbal working memory in treatment-resistant schizophrenia? Am J Psychiatry 154:799–804, 1997

Keverne EB: GABA-ergic neurons and the neurobiology of schizophrenia and other psychoses. Brain Res Bull 48:467–473, 1999

Knoll JL, Garver DL, Ramberg JE, et al: Heterogeneity of the psychoses: is there a neurodegenerative psychosis? Schizophr Bull 24:365–379, 1998

Larsen TK, Opjordsmoen S: Early identification and treatment of schizophrenia: conceptual and ethical considerations. Psychiatry 59:371–380, 1996

Maier W, Lichtermann D, Minges J, et al: Continuity and discontinuity of affective disorders and schizophrenia: results of a controlled family study. Arch Gen Psychiatry 50:871–883, 1993

Marder S, Meibach R: Risperidone in the treatment of schizophrenia. Am J Psychiatry 151:825–835, 1994

Maziade M, Bissonnette L, Rouillard E, et al: 6p24–22 region and major psychoses in the eastern Quebec population. Am J Med Genet (Neuropsychiatr Genet) 74:311–318, 1997

McGorry PD, McFarlane C, Patton GC: The prevalence of prodromal features of schizophrenia in adolescence: a preliminary survey. Acta Psychiatr Scand 92:241–249, 1995

Meehl PE: Schizotaxia revisited. Arch Gen Psychiatry 46:935–944, 1989

Meehl PE: Schizotaxia, schizotypy, schizophrenia. Am Psychol 17:827–838, 1962

Millon T: Classification in psychopathology: rationale, alternatives, and standards. J Abnorm Psychol 100:245–261, 1991

Peralta V, Cuesta MJ: Diagnostic significance of Schneider's first-rank symptoms in schizophrenia. Br J Psychiatry 174:243–248, 1998

Peralta V, Cuesta MJ, Farre C: Factor structure of symptoms in functional psychoses. Biol Psychiatry 42:806–815, 1997

Ratakonda S, Gorman JM, Yale SA, et al: Characterization of psychotic symptoms: use of the domains of psychopathology model. Arch Gen Psychiatry 55:75–81, 1998

Robins E, Guze SB: Establishment of diagnostic validity in psychiatric illness: its application to schizophrenia. Am J Psychiatry 126:983–987, 1970

Rossi A, Mancini F, Stratta P, et al: Risperidone, negative symptoms and cognitive deficit in schizophrenia: an open study. Acta Scand Psychiatr 95:40–43, 1997

Serretti A, Macciardi F, Smeraldi E: Identification of symptomatologic patterns common to major psychoses: proposal for a phenotype definition. Am J Med Genet 67:393–400, 1996

Stip E: The effect of risperidone on cognition in patients with schizophrenia. Can J Psychiatry 41:S35–S40, 1996

Tamminga CA: The promise of new drugs for schizophrenia treatment. Can J Psychiatry 42:265–273, 1997

Tsuang MT, Stone WS, Faraone SV: Schizophrenia: a review of genetic studies. Harv Rev Psychiatry 7:185–207, 1999a

Tsuang MT, Stone WS, Seidman LJ, et al: Treatment of nonpsychotic relatives of patients with schizophrenia: four case studies. Biol Psychiatry 41:1412–1418, 1999b

Tsuang MT, Stone WS, Faraone SV: Toward reformulating the diagnosis of schizophrenia. Am J Psychiatry 157:1041–1050, 2000

Weinberger DR: Schizophrenia as a neurodevelopmental disorder: a review of the concept, in Schizophrenia. Edited by Hirsch SR, Weinberger DR. London, Blackwood Press, 1994

Weinberger DR: Neurodevelopmental perspectives on schizophrenia, in Psychopharmacology: The Fourth Generation of Progress. Edited by Bloom FE, Kupfer DJ. New York, Raven, 1995, pp 1171–1183,

Wildenauer D, Hallmaye RJ, Albus M: A susceptibility locus for affective and schizophrenic disorder? Psychiatr Genet 6:152, 1996

Wildenauer DB, Schwab SG, Maier W, et al: Do schizophrenia and affective disorder share susceptibility genes? Schizophr Res 39:107–111, 1999

Woods BT: Is schizophrenia a progressive neurodevelopmental disorder? toward a unitary pathogenetic mechanism. Am J Psychiatry 155:1661–1670, 1998

Wyatt RJ: Early intervention for schizophrenia: can the course of the illness be altered? Biol Psychiatry 38:1–3, 1995

Index